I Can See Clearly Now

The soundtrack of my life

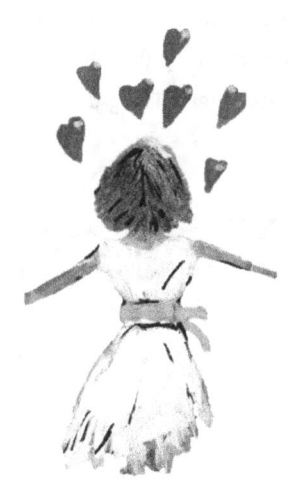

COLLEEN ASHBY

Copyright Notice

 Published by Footprints Publishing, March 2021
© All rights reserved by the author.

This book is copyright. Apart from any fair dealing for the purpose of private study, research, criticism or review, as permitted under the Copyright Act, no part may be reproduced by any process without written permission from the publisher.

Because of the dynamic nature of the Internet, any web addresses or links contained in this book may have changed since publication and may no longer be valid. The views expressed in this work are solely those of the author and do not necessarily reflect the views of the publisher and the publisher hereby disclaims any responsibility for them.

 A catalogue record for this work is available from the National Library of Australia

ISBN (sc): 978-0-6489539-8-2

ISBN (e): 978-0-6489539-9-9

Cover and EXODUS artwork by Heather Kay

Foreword

My name is Patricia Hughes, Colleen Ashby's mother. After I had five boys, Colleen was born in 1964. Her brothers were so happy to have a sister who brought much joy and happiness to the family.

Having older brothers, Colleen was always aiming high to achieve the best in all she undertook. She was swimming by eleven months old and that was just the start of her highly active life.

By the time she was a teenager, horses were her love and she was always looking after them. As soon as she was home from school she was off to her horse, riding, grooming and participating in pony club.

Being a diabetic from age nine was a challenge of a totally different nature. Having to inject herself every day, Colleen learned very quickly to become responsible and independent.

Colleen's diabetes, coupled with her sheer determination to achieve, have been central to the Colleen you will read about in the following pages.

She continues to bring joy and happiness to the whole family and I feel sure you will enjoy reading about her energy, her positive attitude and the challenges she's overcome to be where she is today.

Preface

In 2017 in Perth Western Australia, I had a heart transplant. I am a type 1 diabetic. Type 1 diabetics don't usually get the chance of having a transplant but I am not your normal type 1 diabetic.

When I woke from the operation, I couldn't see. I only had 5% of my sight. Honestly, I'm grateful I still have 5%. I'd have been really pissed off if I'd lost it all. But 5%? I can cope.

So, what makes me grateful? What makes me think I can cope with 5% vision when for most people it would be an insurmountable life event? All my life I've been dealt some tough hands and each time I've just got on with things. Hopefully, the following pages will shed some light into why it is so.

I've been asked to tell the story of my transplant, my road to recovery and the fullness of my life, so that others going through a transplant experience or difficult time, might take something from my journey to help them on theirs.

Here it is.

Colleen Ashby

Contents

Part One

Isn't She Lovely	1
Sugar Sugar	6
Just the Way You Are	10
Better When I'm Dancin'	18
At Last	22
Teach Your Children	25
What a Feeling	30

Part Two

Anyone Who Had a Heart	32
How Can You Mend a Broken Heart	38
Heart of Glass	46
People Get Ready	52
Get Ready for This	58

Part Three

Total Eclipse of the Heart	62
Welcome to My Nightmare	65
I'm Still Standing	129
Breathe	136
Eye of the Tiger	142
Break My Stride	147
Welcome Back	152
Tubthumping	155
Don't Stop Me Now	161

Walking on Sunshine	167
Don't Stop Believin'	174
Ain't No Mountain High Enough	176
Who Let the Dogs Out	181
We Are the Champions	186
Everybody Hurts	191
Father and Daughter	196
Faith	201
Who Are You	206
Here Comes the Sun	209
Turn! Turn! Turn!	211
I Say a Little Prayer	216

PS – I Love You

We Are Family	221

Acknowledgements

Thank You for the Music	225

Finale

What a Wonderful World	229

Author Bio

Part One

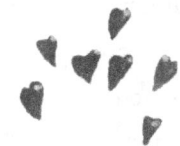

Isn't She Lovely
- Stevie Wonder

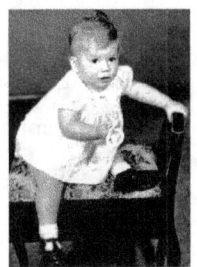

Born in Perth in 1964, the year of the dragon, I was the youngest of six children. Mum and Dad already had five sons: David, Kim, Geoff and twins Will and Eddie, with only eight years between the six of us. Having those older and very protective brothers, I was always safe from anyone who may have wanted to pick on me at school. Eddie and Will were especially protective, even if they heard rumours, so watch out if you were going to give me a hard time. This protectiveness even included my two future husbands being given the brotherly lecture about making sure they did the right thing by their little sis... or else.

If I were asked to describe family life growing up, I would sum it up as 'warm, comfortable and safe' and Mum and Dad were everything a child could want, constant and secure.

Our family life was what, I guess, one might call privileged. Money was never an issue, as my father built a successful agricultural machinery business over thirty years.

Memories of our family life and childhood in Kalamunda in the Perth Hills are

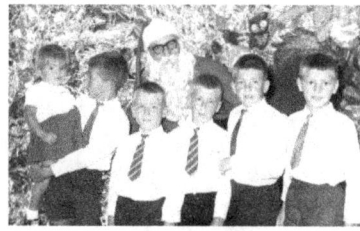 filled with large gatherings, picnics and Christmas parties held at our house, with heaps of wonderful food and our tribe of cousins. Time with my cousins is a particularly heartfelt memory, as we were best of friends during our youth.

Food and treats are a big part of my fond family memories. Friday nights, Dad would drive all us kids to our local deli where we got to choose whatever treats we liked. My favourites were the 2-cent cobbers and the 1-cent milk bottles. A White Knight was also a must have and later on, the Spearmint Knights. Dad's favourite was long liquorice straps and he would buy a box of them to have at home. The boys chose their confectionery and home we would go and all sit together in our large lounge room and watch 'The Flying Nun' on TV. Does it get better than that?

I suppose being the only girl and the youngest, I was 'daddy's little girl.' I have loving memories of a larger than life, teetotal, steady man who made me feel safe.

One memory was of Dad's big, wingback armchair. After Dad's day at work, I would sit up on top of the chair with my legs around his shoulders and I'd comb Dad's short spiky hair while he sat eating apple and cheese. A small memory but one that always gives a warm glow when it comes to mind.

My fondest memory of Dad was this 22 stone, 6-foot 2-inch gentle giant, arms akimbo, legs firm, standing sentry at the end of our pool, the guardian of the water. My brothers and me would take a run towards him and try and push him in the pool. The boys, as they became teenagers, could put up quite a wrestle but they never succeeded in pushing him in. I would take a run at Dad and he would grab my arm and gently fling me off, right up to the other end of the pool, like wiping a fly off his arm. We all loved this game and Dad never gave up until we had all surrendered. Then he would dive in the pool and play with us. Dad always loved his pool time.

Despite running a highly successful agricultural machinery sales company and cattle station, the stories Dad told were always ones from his early days as a policeman in the north of Western Australia. He was a deep and philosophical person. He loved the Aboriginal people from up north very much and respected their gentle ways, their culture and their beliefs. In fact, he respected all cultures and often said if he was closest to any religion, it wasn't the Catholic religion of his birth but more like Buddhism. So, it's not surprising that he was drawn to the spiritual Aboriginal people and right up until his death, this was the narrative that underpinned his life.

My mum was truly a strong woman, with everything she had gone through and dealt with, she was always loving and maternal. Mum supported all her children with whatever we were involved in. If we were part of something, she was there as a parent helper, from Cubs to swimming.

My special time with Mum involved every school holiday during high school. She and I would go down into the city, to Perth, for a week and stay at a hotel. We had a ball ordering room service, going out for meals, going to the pictures and shopping 'till we dropped'. Mum had the 'girl's weekend' thing sorted way back in the 70s and so it's no wonder I enjoy fun times with my girlfriends so much.

I've always had boundless energy and over the years, have dived right into a range of physical sports and pursuits. As children, my brothers and I were all champion swimmers. We even held the local Kalamunda Swimming Club winter swimming training in our large oil-heated pool at home, which had a blow-up igloo over it to keep it warm in the cold months. My brothers all swam competitively into their teenage years, whereas I finished by the time I was eight when, like many young girls, horses became the centre of my life.

I got my first horse when I was six years old and did all the usual horsey things like belonging to a pony club, and later as a teenager, competing in gymkhanas and one day events. Honestly, I breathed, dreamed and talked of nothing but horses throughout my school years. I even dreamed of competing in the Olympics one day.

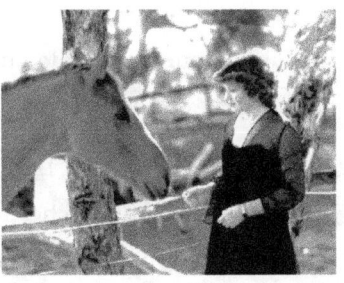

In addition to swimming and horses, ballroom dancing played a significant part of my childhood activities, even working through the various medal levels and participating in dance competitions.

When I was about eight years old, I took up squash. This was another physical activity I loved playing right into my 30s.

Looking back on it, I've always been active, playing a lot of sport but never team sports. Individual sports were the only ones I was ever drawn to or interested in. I guess I never liked the thought of letting the team down if I didn't play well. When you play or compete as an individual, you're the only one you can let down.

While I was charging from one physical activity to the next, inside, my spirituality had started its own journey. My spiritual life has always been a big part of who I am and what motivates me.

As far as I can remember, the journey started when I was 14. Kim had married an astrologer, Margie, and it was from her that I first came to believe we are predestined by our astrological chart. Before we come into our physical life, we choose, our *souls* choose the lessons we need to learn and experience in our lifetime. My spiritual journey makes guest appearances throughout my life and I credit much of my positive outlook to the fact that this is a side of me I have always nurtured and paid attention to.

From where I was standing in 1973, our family life was perfect. But that wasn't the case. When I was around eight years old, Mum left Dad. The boys could choose who they wanted to live with. They went with Dad and Eddie and I moved in with Mum. Dad bought Mum a new house in a suburb of her choosing and the three of us lived there for three or four months. Due to issues that none of us kids found out about until ten or so years later, Mum moved back in with Dad to keep the family together. Eddie and I were back home all together again by November of that year and life seemed back to normal, as far as us kids were concerned.

Mum remained with Dad until I was married. She stayed with Dad to keep the family together until all her babies had flown the nest. That takes a lot of courage. Ten years in a relationship you know you don't want to be in for the sake of your children. That's Mum, always trying to maintain a happy environment for us.

And Mum was there for the boys when all of them, except David, journeyed down the path of drugs and alcohol, mostly smoking dope but Kim and Geoff, at different times, were addicted to heroin. Reaching out to her for help in their time of despair, Mum nursed them through cold turkey in their bedroom for three days on three separate occasions, right through the withdrawals and everything that goes along with it. Always comforting and reassuring them that everything would be alright. She is amazing.

The four boys were heavy dope smokers and when I was about fourteen, the twins talked Mum and me into trying it. Their argument was, Mum needed to try it before she could condemn it, to understand the affects and how safe it really was. That was my first introduction to the world of drugs my brothers were already well acquainted with. Mum and I were shown how to take a toke on the joint, holding it in before blowing it out.

After Mum had pulled on her joint, she became so stoned and lightheaded she had to go and lie down on her bed. She told me afterward she never wanted to try it again and if that was what being stoned was like she wouldn't be able to function properly. As she lay there on the bed, she told me if the house was on fire and burning down, there would be no way she could get up and help save us or herself. She never wanted to be in that predicament again.

I personally didn't get anything from it, nor did I like it but Mum and I had tried it. It wasn't until I was marrying Paul that I tried it again.

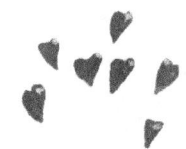

Sugar Sugar
- The Archies

It was during the 1973-74 Christmas holidays, not long after we had all returned home to live with Dad after he and Mum had reconciled, that I began to feel unwell. I was nine years old.

In November, Mum had bought my school uniforms for the new school I was to attend the following year. During the six-week summer holiday, I began dropping weight. I was always fatigued and had an unquenchable thirst. Not only could I not drink enough but I was intensely ravenous, eating all the time. I was getting up five or six times a night to urinate. At first, Mum put it down to the hot summer weather but when I tried on my school uniform at the beginning of term, it just hung off me. I had lost a stone in weight and for a nine-year-old who wasn't overweight to begin with, that was an extreme weight loss in a short amount of time.

Mum made a doctor's appointment two weeks from the start of school and on Valentine's Day, I was diagnosed with diabetes, ending up in hospital that afternoon.

Two weeks in Princess Margaret hospital learning how to give myself injections and how to test my urine for blood glucose levels, along with learning the diet and portion control of carbohydrates and 'free' foods like proteins, was all part of the new regime that was to be my life from that point on.

In those days, Mum would have to boil up the glass syringe and reusable needles, the gauge or width of those needles were like horse injections and they would get blunt after several uses. I remember sitting on the edge of my bed in the mornings, injection drawn up in my hand, pausing reluctantly, not wanting to stick that thing into either my legs or stomach. Needle hovering, taunting me with its inevitable sting waiting to be inflicted upon me. Sometimes I think I was there suspended in what seemed an eternity, or at least five minutes, before being brave enough to commit myself to the almighty dread of the needle going in.

I remember teaching my cousin, Sharon, how to test my wee. I would wee in a potty, then take five drops of urine, ten drops of water and in with the clini-test tablet. It would bubble and fizz all the way up the test tube until it calmed down and turned into a colour. Blue meant there was no sugar in the urine (a hypo glycaemic event, shaky, sweaty and feeling wobbly, would normally be felt). A green colour indicated the sugar level was low, ranging up through about three more colours. The highest was bright orange and that meant you had way too much sugar in your body. Between you and me, I quite often had orange-coloured wee tests but please don't tell anyone.

I've been through all the changes in technological advancements for diabetes. From boiled glass syringes and large needles to the first disposable syringes then the amazing insulin pens. Today I have a CBM, a Constant Blood-glucose Monitoring device. You inject a tiny hair-like wire into yourself which stays in one spot for a week. It has a small computer chip connected to it and is then Bluetoothed to your mobile phone. You enter all the details of food, insulin and exercise and anytime you need to know your blood sugar level, it's right there at your fingertips all the time. Truly amazing and so much easier.

But there were things going on in my body I couldn't see. In my 20s, an endoscopy confirmed I had Coeliac Disease, so that gave me another dietary regime I have always had trouble sticking too. With gluten, I could always cheat a little bit with no dire consequences, except for farting like a brewery horse and bloating like a sheep that needs a good knee jabbed into its guts. I did come to realise the internal damage was always occurring but as I couldn't see it, I guess I didn't really take it seriously.

Thankfully, gluten free products have improved in 20 years and you'll be pleased to know, I do look after my coeliac a lot better as I've got older.

In all, I know I had a privileged childhood, despite having type 1 diabetes. Having diabetes never stopped me from doing anything. Both Mum and Dad always believed in letting me live life to the full. I continued horse riding, squash and doing all the normal things other kids did.

I never even thought having diabetes should make any difference to being able to participate in life fully, like anyone else, and I never made a fuss about it and quite often didn't tell people I had it. Why did I need to? I knew how to control it and I took care of my own injections; it was no big deal.

Looking back, I do think I rebelled, as most teenagers do when they are dealt a health issue like diabetes that makes them different and sets them apart from their peers. When other kids would eat lollies or eat junk food, I didn't want to be different and would consume whatever they were having. No one likes to be different from their peers and I was no exception.

With a fairly ordinary, comfortable suburban Australian upbringing behind me, I emerged as a young adult, confident and happy, despite the daily reminder of type 1 diabetes.

Contrast that with some of my brothers who went down the path of drug and alcohol dependency. Why? Why them and not me? We all grew up in the same home, with the same parents. What was it about me that made me shine when life threw up challenges? Why did my inner voice say, 'You can do it. Don't give up. Do your best. Keep on trying.'

Perhaps there are a couple of things at work here. I was the youngest child of six. Did I compete with five older boys? Yes. As the only girl, was I spoiled? Yes. Did I grow up feeling safe and secure, knowing I could do anything? Absolutely. Was I given heaps of opportunities? Yes.

I really think it's that cradle of safety, love, support and devotion, from not just Mum and Dad but all my protective brothers that has contributed to my positive 'can do' attitude to life. Thank you, universe for the accident of my birth and this gift of positivity you bestowed on me throughout my life.

There's no doubt diabetes, despite being a pain in the arse, has taught me to 'get over it and get on with it.' Yes, there were times when I dearly wished I didn't have this thing hanging over me, day in day out but now I can see that it's been a gift. A gift of patience, perseverance and acceptance of 'the way things are.'

Just the Way You Are
– Billy Joel

I was 16 in 1981 when I met Paul, my future husband, at our family's New Year's Eve party. He was friends with my family during the swimming club years, so the reunion with our family was easy. When we met at that New Year's Eve party, he was in the navy and had to go back to Sydney in a week's time. He asked me to go out with him on New Year's Day and we spent the rest of that week going out together, enjoying each other's company. We decided to write to each other until he could get home again and then, just like that, at the end of our week together, he was gone.

Keeping true to our promise, I wrote to Paul every day and he wrote almost the same. He said he loved it when the men received mail, as some guys may get one or two letters, others none, then there was him, with a pile the other blokes envied.

Paul returned to Perth six weeks later for a funeral and so we got to see one another again. I remember hearing his big V8 Monaro arrive at the family home like it was yesterday. I went outside and there he was, like a scene out of 'An Officer and a Gentleman'. 6 ft tall and handsome, striding towards me in full white officer's uniform and cap. He was quite literally my knight in shining

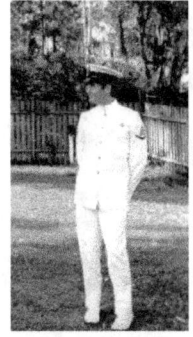
armour, truly sweeping me off my feet. No girl could ask for a more romantic encounter. That was it, I was hooked.

We spent that week going out when I got home from school, I was in year 12 (my final high school year) and Paul would pick me up in front of the Catholic girl's college I was attending. Man, I loved that. Making everybody look as I got into his bright yellow V8.

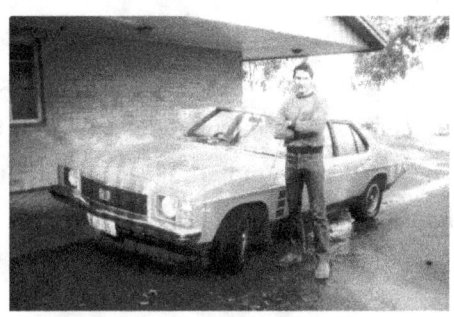

It was only a few days after he got back to Sydney that he called me, after he had spoken to Mum first, and asked me to marry him. My simple response was, 'Yeah. OK then,' and with that, I was engaged at 16 and still at school. We actually didn't get married until I was 19 and that's an interesting story in itself.

Paul and I, or should I say, my parents, had planned a large formal wedding. Horse and carriage, guests from the business and all our relatives. It was going to be a grand wedding indeed. Invitations had been printed and venues booked. However, due to a misunderstanding with not having children at the wedding, a family member on Paul's side got their nose out of joint. Long story short, family feuding began and soon neither of his parents were coming to the wedding. Stress was now at a high level, so I cancelled the whole thing. The only way out of this huge mess was to get rid of it and that is what I did. I then moved out of home and when the shit had finally settled from hitting the fan, I revisited the idea. This time, though, Paul and I planned a small ceremony with only immediate siblings and parents. Thirty people was the much-reduced number from one hundred and seventy. At least it was a wedding we had planned and were in control of and not some huge glamorous wedding event of the year.

It was 1983 when we eventually married and we built our house in the Perth Hills on a shared, thirty-acre property with my brother David and his wife Gail. A driveway halved the property, David on one side and Paul and I on the other.

Paul and I were happy building our nest; building stables, clearing paddocks and constructing a dressage arena and a few jumps for me to work my horses. I loved it out there in the water catchment forest area in the hills, with numerous, gorgeous trails and dirt tracks to ride my horses.

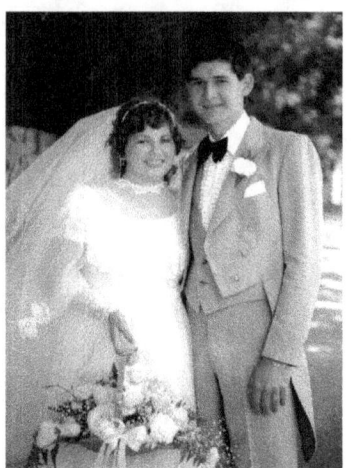

The only thing I didn't always like were the kangaroos, especially when they would be standing still in the bush and then suddenly take off. This usually guaranteed a spooked horse. Startled by the kangaroo, the horse would jump suddenly which meant, nine times out of ten, I would end up thrown off the horse and on the ground. That wasn't the worst of it. Worse was the long trek back home on foot because the horse would have run back home, waiting patiently for me at the gate.

Paul was never really a horse rider but I managed to get him on a horse a few times and we went on a few lovely trail rides together. It was a happy union for the first seven years of being together but the arrival of our child saw my vision of enjoying family life evaporate before my eyes.

Paul and my brothers were close friends and my brothers had soon introduced him to the habit of smoking dope. It didn't really bother me, Paul smoking, pulling his bongs either by himself or with my brothers, who were regular visitors. As I said, I was happy doing my own things. I would either do an aerobics class after work or be out riding my horses. I could count on two hands the amount of times I pulled a bong with Paul and my brothers over the seven years of marriage and they were well before I was pregnant with our son Stephen.

Saying I was happy doing my own thing was true but deep down I was pissed off with how much Paul smoked and drank. I hated going out to functions, as I would be the one trying to drag him away from the last dregs of beer in the jugs left on the table. His drinking was becoming more of a problem, too but I guess I naïvely thought once we had kids this would all magically just disappear. Still young and with not enough worldly knowledge of how these habits are hard to get rid of, I just had to get on enjoying my life in my own way, while Paul enjoyed his.

Paul and I did, on several occasions, discuss the matter of when we had children, his drinking and pot smoking would not be part of family life. Paul had always agreed he would give it up when we had kids.

And so, the arrival in 1989 of our beautiful boy, Stephen, was deeply joyous for both me and Paul. Paul was so proud to have a son. For me, of course, I loved him from the moment he was born, as I did all our boys.

But there was an added poignancy to Stephen's arrival and the reason Mum had such a special connection with him. At some stage during my childhood, I found out my brother before me, Stephen, had drowned in our backyard swimming pool. I secretly decreed I would name my first-born son in memory of him, for Mum. As the universe would have it in its full magnificence, my Stephen was even born on the same date as Mum's Stephen. It felt good that I could gift Mum something so poignant and meaningful. It seemed the gods were working to make this so for Mum. It really was meant to be.

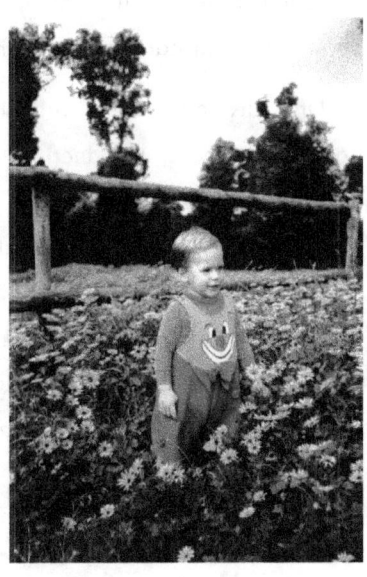

Our marriage went by so smoothly up until the birth of Stephen, because as I've alluded to, we were, in many ways, both living our own separate lives. That works, of course, until the status changes. Having a baby certainly changes the way you intend to live your life. It may mean having to give up comforts or habits you enjoy. Paul had tried to reduce his drinking and smoking but he just couldn't make the change and give up those vices.

Stephen was 12 months old when I found the clarity and strength I needed to end the marriage once and for all, through an incredible transformational experience.

My brother, Eddie, introduced me to my first encounter of a personal higher self-awareness workshop. Eddie had already done the workshop and afterwards, was on such a super-high charge of energy and positivity, I thought, 'I want to get some of that.'

In the workshop, I learned about creative visualisation, how to recall memory items quickly and how we can access more of our mind to create the reality we want. I felt more self-assertive and empowered and was beginning to see the world in a different way. Practicing the techniques every day, I began to know the power of my mind.

A few months later, a follow-up weekend workshop was announced and I booked it. Paul had Stephen for the weekend while I did the workshops.

Off I drove to the beautiful, forested place in Jarrahdale where cabins and dormitories were built deep into the wooded landscape. Over the weekend, we did meditations, learned about our higher consciousness and how we are programmed by our parenting, schooling, society and the community surrounding us. A journey of self-discovery and delving into the aspects of ourselves, our fears and beliefs that were not true to ourselves. Fears and beliefs about ourselves we needed to let go. The culmination of all this work was to be a walk across burning coals by each participant.

On the Sunday, a large fire pit was built and lit, so by night fall there would be a path of glowing red-hot coals for each of us to walk over. We each wrote down the things we wanted to let go, then in a procession, we were to walk up to the fire to renounce our burdens and walk across the glowing embers. To prepare for the fire walk and so we didn't suffer burns, we first meditated on how to visualise a cool surface like snow, water or grass. My mantra for walking on the hot coals was, 'cool green grass, cool green grass.' And then, to charge our personal energy, together in a large room with music blaring, all of us danced vigorously to increase our energy. We were now ready to prove the conviction of the power of the mind.

Walking towards the firepit in the dark, amongst a group of energetically charged people, was both exciting and disconcerting at the same time. Now was the time for the ultimate test of the power of our minds. We really *could* walk across hot coals with just the power of our mind and get across unharmed.

As I walked towards the fire, I was struggling to overcome the immense fear that kept encroaching into my mind telling me I couldn't do it. What the hell made me think I was capable of walking on burning coals? It takes years of practice to be able to do this sort of stuff. 'I'm not going to do it. I don't want to get my feet burned. No way.' This was the voice rattling loudly in my head.

Reaching the intense heat and fiery red glow of this mesmerising fire pit, it was now so real. Fear was escalating inside of me and as I watched a few people make their journey across the burning abyss, I knew deep down I had to do it. I had to know for myself if I had it in me. I at least had to try or else this weekend had been a waste.

Walking up to the pit, my heart was pounding in my chest. The instructor told me to breathe, close my eyes and get my visualisation in my head and when I was ready, I could take my first step into self-empowerment. Ready with my visualization and mantra, 'cool green grass,' I repeated the mantra over and over in my head. Visualizing a field of beautiful, cool, rich green grass before me, I took my first step. Keeping focus on this picture in my mind, I didn't think about the intense heat under my feet. I didn't even feel the heat at all, only the 'cool green grass' I was walking on.

Reaching the other side, the instructor grabbed my hand and hugged me. Realising what I had just done, I broke out in waves of sobs. Tears flooded from my eyes and in my chest, uncontrollable waves of emotion and adrenalin took over. Once he let go, a feeling of empowerment, strength and self-realisation rose inside me and I felt invincible.

There were several people who did get their feet burned quite badly. Losing focus halfway across and not believing they could do it but doing it anyway. Some had to be carried back as they couldn't walk on their burned feet. For me, however, it was the most empowering thing I have ever done and would be the catalyst that would create my positive and creative journey for the rest of my life.

Driving home that night feeling exhilarated and beyond anything I have felt before, I knew then the marriage with Paul was not heading in the direction I had envisioned for having a family. I knew too I was the only one who could change it and do something about it. It's no good wishing for something but not taking any action towards it. A motto that was to become a mantra of mine for living was, 'life rewards action.' You can talk the talk but until you take the first step, that's all it will ever be, talk.

Home again and settling back into family life with Stephen, now 16 months old, I wrote Paul a letter saying how I felt and that the life I wanted as a family and the behaviours of his drinking and smoking dope was not what we had agreed on once children came along.

Leaving the letter for him to read, I booked into a motel for two nights with Stephen to give Paul time to think about my needs and his. What was he was willing to compromise on? Was he willing to give up his vices for our family life?

Over the next couple of months, Paul tried at first to modify his behaviour and cut down the drinking and smoking pot but it didn't last and he soon reverted to his consumption of at least a six pack of beers a night plus the dope. So, I made the call and ended the relationship. Now don't get me wrong, making that decision was not easy or without a lot of stress, self-doubt and fear for the future but I knew the situation I was in was not serving me in happiness and I wanted more than that, so I had to close the door on that part of my life.

I don't lay blame on anyone here; we all have choices in our lives and we are the ones responsible for them. Once a choice is made, then you must live with it and move on and hopefully grow from the lesson learnt. If life was all rainbows and lollypops, then no learning would ever be had. We only truly learn from our mistakes and life's challenges, so we need to acknowledge the lessons they teach us.

Here again comes my streak of resilience. Why is it I can face up to the truth of a situation, accept my part in it and make the change? I know many people have trouble seeing the truth or seeing clearly the situation they are in. And when you are in a situation, boy it's hard to see it for what it really is.

If you can see clearly while you are mired in the muck, the next step is seeing your contribution to where you find yourself. If you have the courage, and it takes heaps of courage, to face up to the part you've played, then you have the courage for the next step and that is to make a change.

If I'm honest, I went in with eyes wide open and married the tall, handsome officer in the uniform with the awesome car without much thought to 'ever after'. When 'ever after' started to unfold, I drew on something deep inside and found the courage to make the change I needed to, for my son's sake and for my happiness.

I thank my lucky stars, as well as my resilience, that I'm a person that says 'yes' to life and opportunity. Seeing my brother so pumped after he'd done the creative visualisation workshop made me curious, made me want some of that. Would I have left Paul as quickly and decisively as I did had I not gone to the workshops? Probably, but it would have taken longer, I have no doubt. Would I have even thought of going to a visualisation workshop if I hadn't already keyed into my spiritual side? Perhaps not.

Looking back at this time, I think my resilience, which I believe largely stems from living with this annoying and ever-present disease, type 1 diabetes, and being in touch with my spiritual side, were really important for helping me see the situation as it was, the truth of it, despite being very difficult and then accepting my part in it and having the courage to change.

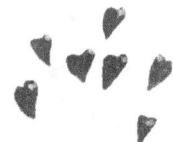

Better When I'm Dancin'
– Meghan Trainor

Well, like most people left from the wreckage of a marriage, I looked for things to do and ways to perhaps meet another knight in shining armour. And if he could ballroom dance, all the better.

Dancing turned out to be the saviour of my life. And like everything I turned my hand to, I dived in and was totally passionate about it. I went through the medal levels again, with social dancing three to four nights a week. I met a lot of wonderful people who became a wonderful social group.

Every couple of weeks on a Saturday night, we would all go to a social dance function, always relaxed and comfortable with each other. I met my dear girlfriend, Sue, through dancing and right up to this day, she has remained a close part of my life. We were dance partners in crime, playing tricks by doing some swapping moves in the progression dances, completely confusing the men. It was the best seven years of my life. Even today, I reminisce fondly about those days.

There was one partner I used to dance with regularly and felt totally at ease talking to him on any subject or matter and of course, he was also a very competent dancer, which was of the upmost importance. He had a daughter who had type 1 diabetes, so knew the obvious symptoms of a hypo or low blood sugar level. When he asked me for a dance, I would jump up straight away eager to hit the dance floor but within minutes he would tell me to sit down and eat some jellybeans. Being stubborn and cantankerous, a common sign of hypoglycaemia, I would say, 'No, I'm alright.' Starting to get shaky, jumbling my words and not making any sense, he would make me sit down and eat something sugary. No hiding or getting away with any symptoms from him, which was most probably a good thing. Sometimes I could be too stubborn for my own good. I still wouldn't let the diabetes make an impact on my life. It would have to fit in around me.

I think one of my underlying romantic Libran dreams was to find a new life partner who would dance me off my feet, get married and have a couple of children. Stephen was still only four and young enough to just settle into a new family life. I dreamt my husband would be a great dancer and we would regularly go to dances and show off the smooth grooves and moves that comes with dancing together over time. If the house and the proverbial white picket fence came into the equation, that would be a bonus I could certainly live with quite contentedly.

In this dance partner, I thought I had found Mr Right. I was besotted with him. I was 30 and he was 55. I always liked older men. They seemed to have a sense of understanding and more worldly knowledge, so perhaps I thought an older man would look after me, keep me safe and secure? He told me he loved talking and being around me as I was the most refreshing person he had ever known. I didn't quite know what he meant by that and I took it as a compliment. I went out with him and his kids and took Stephen too. I imagined an already made instant family but he only ever wanted friendship and dancing while I was envisioning wedding bells.

When I was about to head off to Canada on a trip to visit my dad, filled with trepidation and uncertainty of what might lay ahead, I told him my fears about leaving. He told me it would be a great adventure and to do it. Deep down inside, I was hoping he would romantically tell me not to leave and to stay with him. But that was only my romantic Libran imagination.

So heartbroken, I went on my adventure to Canada. Stephen and I were going to stay with my dad and his second wife, Ellie Mae. Dad flew us there and we could stay with him for as long as we wanted.

We spent four months with Dad travelling 20,000 kms all around British Columbia, Alberta, Saskatchewan, Montana and Idaho. It was the most amazing time going off road to rural areas of the country. It was a time of exploration and learning new things. It was also a brave adventure on my part. Even though I had done a lot of overseas travel with Mum all through my younger years, going somewhere different every year, I was now by myself with a four-year-old and baggage.

I wrote all the time to my dance partner telling of my adventures and drawing pictures on his letters and envelopes to show how much he meant to me. But I was also hoping to meet my romantic Canadian Mounty who would sweep me off my feet. This would resolve the heartbreak I was dealing with.

When I did finally return, we met up and he said he loved reading all my letters and the drawings but he knew I had a different notion to what he had. He told me he was seeing another woman and a relationship was never on the cards for us; he just enjoyed my refreshing company. With that, we never really danced together anymore.

So while I never found my prince charming on the ballroom floor, I made some wonderful connections, which was an integral part of my life at that time.

Around this time, my cousin Sharon had come to live with me after she returned from working abroad and needed somewhere to live. I told Sharon she could stay in my house while Stephen and I were away in Canada and then see what happened down the track. After four months in Canada, Stephen and I returned and Sharon decided to stay on living with us and from that time, we have an extremely close connection with each other.

We nicknamed each other 'Hon'. There was a scene from 'Cat Woman' where Michelle Pfeiffer comes home and on walking through her front door says, 'Hi Honey, I'm home.' Then there is a pause, there is no response and she sadly announces, 'Oh, that's right, I live alone.' That's what Sharon would announce when she arrived home from work and so that became our catch phrase. Since then, we've called each other 'Hon.'

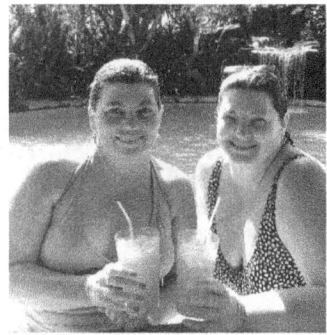

For eight years, when Hon moved down to live and work in Margaret River, she became 'Southern Hon' and I was 'Northern Hon'. That's how we would sign our Birthday and Christmas cards to each other.

Even just recently, while getting our eyebrows done, the beautician only found out Sharon's name wasn't Hon when she was making a booking. It's just automatic now and doesn't feel right if we call each other by our first names. We don't even care if people might think we are a lesbian couple, that just makes things more fun.

One day, when Hon was still living with me, we heard this loud clanging noise coming from the church next door to us. Walking over to see what the loud noise was, we were introduced to the amazing world of clogging. Not Dutch style clogging but flat lace-up shoes with a metal tap in the toe and heel of the shoe which came from the Appalachian Mountains. Initially, it was a cowboy dance that has progressed into being performed with modern pop music.

We joined the group and had the time of our lives clogging away together. I eventually took over running the 'Gumnut Cloggers' in Kalamunda, leaving the ballroom far behind me.

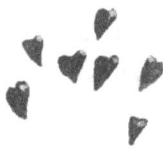

At Last
– Etta James

I've mentioned my amazing school holiday treats staying in a city hotel with Mum and how much fun that was. Fast forward to my adult years and some of my fondest memories are of times spent with Hon and my good friend, Sue. Great music, eating, drinking and very importantly, playing Canasta for sheep stations.

Our close friendship included us giving each other special titles, as befitting our special place in each other's esteem. Hon's alias was 'Goddess', a self-appointed moniker she had since growing up in her family. Sue gave me the title 'Precious' due to my sensitivity to light, noise and comfort. Such was my sensitivity; I would have to get aluminium foil and tape it to the window to block out the smallest glint of light. The smallest glint would wake me up in the mornings and prevent me from falling asleep. It was the same with noise at night. Beds too had to be 'just right'. With that in mind, because we already had a 'Goddess' I became a 'Princess', my full title being, 'Princess Precious'. So, what title for Sue? Somewhat bewildered as to the correct title Hon and I could bestow upon her, we knew she couldn't be a 'Queen', as that would make her higher than me and that was not happening. Hon came up with the title 'Duchess'. Yes, that was a fitting title indeed. Just 'Duchess' though? Surely she should have a full title. The full title was obvious and came from the bouts of Tourette's-like explosions that erupted while Sue participated in our games of Canasta. Sue would come out with a loud, 'F**k,' with a slight pause before pronouncing, 'ola.' Obviously, she was 'Duchess F**k Ola' but for the sake of good taste in the presence of others, she was merely 'Duchess Ola'.

We shared some very funny, R-rated language and slightly intoxicated games of Canasta on our girl's getaway at Hon's place. Canasta was a game requiring at least an hour and a half to play and of course you needed to play the best of three rounds to announce the final champion. So, as you can see, we needed a bit of time to fulfil our serious commitment to the art of playing Canasta. Personally, I think Canasta should be included in the Olympics, or at least up there in a chess championship-type of tournament. I'm quite sure we would all be crowned champions.

Meanwhile, in amongst the ballroom dancing, clogging and boozy Canasta weekends, I was bringing up Stephen along with the support of Mum who was an absolute brick, as she had always been.

Stephen's first eight years of he and I being together was one of pure devotion; all my love and time was spent on him. With Mum always present and Hon in the year that she lived with us, he was always surrounded by feminine, nurturing love. Stephen had our undivided attention.

Stephen was a happy little boy with all that love and attention. He was an avid tee-ball player, competing in the inter-district games as well. I loved being a third base coach and practice throwing and catching with him. It was a favourite pastime.

But despite all his love and attention and despite thriving at school and with sport and other activities, Stephen yearned for a constant father figure. Each year when he sat on Santa's knee in the shopping centre, he asked for a dad for Christmas. My heartbreaking memory of him will always be watching this little boy sitting up on our brick letterbox on a Sunday morning, waiting for his dad to collect him on his access visit. Paul was always late but Stephen just sat and waited, often for well over an hour, and wouldn't come in until his dad arrived. Seeing this little boy waiting patiently for this incredibly important person in his life still gives me a feeling of great sadness.

Like others before him in the family, drugtaking and alcohol abuse eventually consumed Stephen's life. Something that has devastated me and I carry with me every day. Whether it's something in our genetic makeup that draws us to drug and alcohol addiction or whether in the case of Stephen, his addictions stem from his own personal journey and issues regarding a father figure, I will never know. Perhaps it's a combination of both. Most probably it is...

I met my second husband, Les, in the local television repair shop when I had to get my radio fixed. Well, that's not exactly correct. What happened was, our family friend Wendy had an electrical repair shop and had a new guy working for her. He'd recently returned from fifteen years in America, having split with his wife and leaving three girls behind. Wendy told Mum she thought Les and I would get on and so between them, they arranged for me to take Mum's radio in for repair on a day that no one else would be in the shop. Yep, it was a set up.

Knowing the score, I went in and started a conversation with this complete stranger. We spoke for about 15 minutes and the following week I went to collect the radio and gave him my phone number. He phoned me the next night and we have never looked back. So, there you go. No officer's uniform, no horse, no ballroom glitter, just a good and handsome man in a local television repair shop.

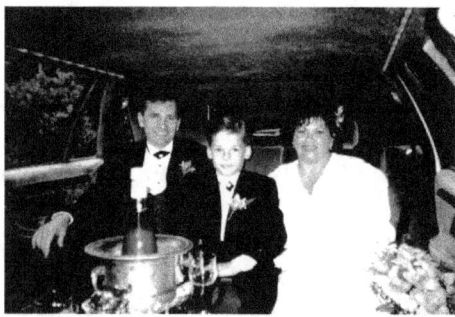

The funny thing is, Les never knew about this set up until about five years ago.

Les and I were married eight months later. Stephen was only eight years old and saw Les as a new dad to have around, even though Stephen was still seeing and connecting with Paul.

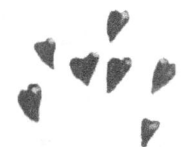

Teach Your Children
– Crosby, Stills and Nash

Not long after we were married, I fell pregnant and it was a girl. I was so excited as I had always wanted a little girl. With all those brothers, I'd had a lifetime of men. A girl would be a nice change.

At the 19-week scan, they picked up an anomaly and after having an amniocentesis performed, I was told she had no middle section of her heart and aborting her now was the best solution. Heartbroken, Les and I went and saw a paediatric cardiologist for a second opinion. He explained there was a 5% chance that if we got her to 24 weeks, there was a chance of flying her to Melbourne to have heart surgery. I told him he gave us 5% more chance than the obstetrician and I would take that 5% of hope. Thanking him, we left with a tiny glimmer of hope.

When I went back to the hospital for another scan, they picked up that she had died in utero. I was induced and gave birth to our beautiful little Beth. Stephen, Mum and Les all got to hold her over the next few days that I was in hospital, making funeral arrangements at the same time.

At the funeral, I was finding it hard to keep myself together but when I saw my twin brothers carrying Beth's tiny white coffin up on their shoulders as pall bearers, I burst out crying. I was completely heartbroken.

An autopsy had shown some of Beth's organs were around the wrong way, so even if the heart could have been fixed, she would have had a lot of health issues regardless.

Poor little Stephen had to contend with the death of his little sister-to-be. I was so consumed by grief myself and never really thought about how he was dealing with it, he never showed any signs of showing his emotions. Looking back, I realise how resilient children are but deep down, they are truly affected. I'm sorry, Stephen, for not being better for you during that time of crisis.

After swimming again with my girlfriend Sue, we talked over coffee. Sue said to me I may have another chance of having a girl. My quick and intuitive answer was, 'No, that was the only chance of having a girl.' It was just my gut feeling and I stated it quite factually; it was an inner knowing.

Some months later, I fell pregnant and another time of excitement was in our grasp. I was feeling positive about the pregnancy and at a 12-week scan after I had started spotting, it turned out to be an ectopic pregnancy. That was the end of that.

Now, wavering thoughts of whether a successful pregnancy would ever occur were starting to taunt my mind. I knew having diabetes, especially type 1, is always classified as high risk, let alone I was now 34 years old.

I was still doing my clogging and life carried on with Stephen at primary school and playing tee ball and us still being a happy family. Then I became pregnant again but not telling anyone this time until I was past the 12-week mark and everything had checked out OK. Finally, I was able to start telling family and friends we were pregnant. At the dreaded 19-week scan, I was told I was having a very healthy boy. Relieved and extremely happy, everything was finally on track. I ran the 'Gumnut Cloggers' until I was 32 weeks pregnant with Scott, then I gave it up. I had also been swimming with my girlfriend Sue during this whole pregnancy to keep fit and healthy.

I was admitted to hospital at 32 weeks with pre-eclampsia, which was the same with Stephen all those years before. Knowing my history, however, the doctors weren't going to risk me sitting in hospital waiting for things to start going wrong, so I gave birth to Scott by caesarean section at 35 weeks.

Les was so excited to have another child of his own. He had three girls from his previous marriage and they were all in America. A little boy was exactly what was needed and Stephen had a little brother. We also let Stephen choose all the middle names of his siblings, which he loved doing.

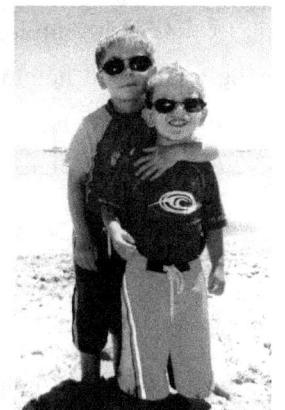

Everything was going along smelling like roses. We built a new home and moved in when Scott was six weeks old. Working on the new home was an ongoing project we all loved doing. I fell pregnant again and as per Stephen and Scott's pregnancies, I was admitted at 34 weeks and at 36 weeks our gorgeous Mark arrived into our family.

All pregnancies, except for Beth, were caesareans. Part of having diabetes from childhood is that bone structures don't form properly so my pelvis was like that of a 12-year-old. Caesareans were my only option for a full-term baby. Just an interesting little fact I thought I'd add in.

Ten years between Stephen and Scott and 18 months between Scott and Mark. Stephen loved having two little brothers to play with and to teach.

I had always been a stay-at-home mum, just like I was raised. I felt it was my place to be at home looking after the children. I had made that decision right from my first marriage. Prior to the birth of Stephen, I worked for five years putting all our earnings into paying off the mortgage, going without floor coverings, insulation in the ceiling, painting or window coverings. Literally putting every cent we made on the mortgage. We managed to pay it off in five years and during the year I fell pregnant, got all the comfortable items put into the house. Then it felt right to stay at home and be with the children.

By the time we had Scott and Mark, Mum lived on the same block as us, so a close 'nanna' relationship was enjoyed by all three boys. Mum was a very interactive nanna. Reading, painting, cooking, gardening and letting them make a mess and enjoy their time with her exploring the world around them. Picnics, outings and family holidays were always enjoyed with Nanna. She was an integral part of our loving extended family. Mum would do kindy rosters, reading to other children in the school and has always been a very active part of our children's lives, including running Stephen to tee-ball training if I was busy with Scott and Mark. She always made her love available to the boys. Even when they were going for their driver's licence, she would let them drive her car everywhere to get the hours required to obtain a licence. Now she is older, all those years of baby sitting and helping with the children are being returned. We now help her out around the house doing things she can no longer do for herself. Our intergenerational living arrangement has made for a wonderful and enriched life for us all.

Life was moving on, you know how it is with kids, a treadmill in many ways and for us with three young boys, it was full on.

In 2005, I was helping at Scott's kindy and by the time pre-primary came around, the principal at the school suggested I did The Educational Assistants course, as she thought I would make a good one. I did just that.

One year later, I had my Certificate 4 Special Needs Educational Assistant qualification. My plan was to be able to be at the same school as my children and be there for them if they needed me. Both Scott and Mark had been diagnosed as being on the Autism Spectrum and not surprisingly, I had a personal and passionate interest in this area.

I was fascinated to learn the brain can be physically hardwired differently to that of a neuro-typical brain. Once you understand the logic and reasoning of the brain processing of someone with Autism, you understand they are truly the most amazing and brilliant, caring and kind people. My first-hand experience with working and living with someone on the autism spectrum showed me if they are given the right support and understanding and allowed to follow their 'special interest' then they become the most productive, beautiful and intriguing adults.

Any parent who has had a child or, as in our case, two children diagnosed with a disability, will know what Les and I went through when we first learned of their diagnoses. I remember leaving the doctor's rooms and going to a café with Les. We just sat and cried. At the time we didn't know why we were crying; yes we were shocked but looking back, I know now we were crying for the life our boys would never have. We were crying for all the things we thought they would do, all the plans we had for them. We were grieving. Grieving for the lives the boys were not going to live. Everything had to change. Our expectations, our understanding of the boys and their ways. We knew we needed to put our expectations aside and now look forward to providing the best life and opportunities for the boys possible.

Once again, my resilience and determination, and Les's, also came to the fore and we pivoted on the spot, recalibrated our expectations and focused our energies on understanding the boys and building on their strengths.

Of course, I was afraid for them and at times, overwhelmed for them making their way in the world once they had finished their education. But mine and Les's determination to understand and develop their strengths and innate abilities was stronger than our doubts and fears.

Les shone in this respect. He keyed into the boy's natural strengths and yes, in some cases, obsessions, and worked with the boys hands on, without a textbook in sight, to foster their interests. For Mark, it was mechanics and how things worked. For Scott, it was technology and computers.

The boys didn't know they had a diagnosis of autism for a very long time. Both Les and I didn't want them to use their diagnosis as an excuse not to try, succeed or excel in any way. This worked for us and for them. They are disciplined and hard working. They are extremely competent in their fields of endeavour and have secured full-time employment. I couldn't ask for more.

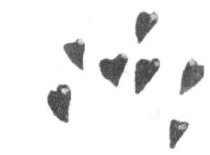

What a Feeling
– Irene Cara

By 2005 I had become a real gym junkie, participating in aerobic classes and doing strength training. At the end of the year of completing my Certificate 4, the aerobics instructor said to me, 'You should do your Certificate in Fitness Instruction, you would be a great instructor.' Well that was the brightest light bulb moment I'd had up to that point. Totally excited with the idea of being up there on stage instructing a group of people, working out to music, Yeah Baby.

I spent 2006 obtaining my Cert. 4 in Fitness Instruction and Personal Training. I absolutely loved it. I was by far the oldest in the course, with most of the students just finishing high school and some didn't even have their licence yet. I was 42 years old and so told the kids to just call me 'Mum.' It was great and I related so well with them, helping them with their confidence and providing reassurance that everything would be OK and not to stress about doing things in front of people.

That was the beginning of the next best three years of my life. I was working at four different gyms, doing aerobics, personal training, boot camps, gym appraisals and writing programs for clients. I loved it. Averaging 14 aerobic classes per week, man I was on fire and extremely fit. I couldn't get enough of that endorphin rush that hits you about ten minutes into the workout. I always have, and still do, find the warmup the hardest slog while your body is starting its pre-check and firing up the different systems inside. Crank up the music and man, I was away. I was a real 80s music fan and would occasionally throw in a bit of 70s disco sounds, something most people could sing along to. I was in my element being up there in front of a group, inspiring, having fun and motivating people. That was definitely my 'thing.'

I also had a contract at the primary school which fitted in with the fitness work, so I had the best of both worlds. Being there at school with my kids and fitting in the gym around that. Life was good.

In September 2009, I had to have shoulder surgery due to too much resistance training. Yep, I'd over done it and I had broken my acromion, which is the bone on the top of the shoulder. It had to be pinned and wired. Surgery wasn't an issue for me because over the past six years or so, I had all my trigger fingers (joints locking), both wrists, carpal tunnels and frozen or encapsulated left shoulder operated on. All part and parcel of long-term diabetic complications. Nothing worth mentioning. This was just another surgery I had to get done.

During recovery of the right pinned shoulder, it froze as well and even under anaesthetic the surgeon couldn't manipulate it. It was a long twelve months of being a couch potato without being able to use my arm. I still worked at the primary school and so life continued for our busy family.

I know for some elite sports men and women and those with the endorphin addiction, which I obviously had, when faced with a significant injury which takes them away from their life blood, it's the beginning of significant depression and self-doubt. For me, it wasn't. Once again, my resilience and positive attitude seemed to click into gear. So I couldn't do the exercise I once did but I was busy with the boys and attending to their needs, the exercise could take a break, which it did until 2011.

Part Two

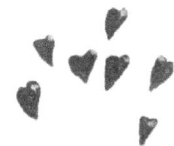

Anyone Who Had a Heart
– Dionne Warwick

In 2011, I decided I had to get my fitness back. Enough of sitting around waiting for movement and rotation of my arm to happen. I could go back to teaching 'spin' classes, which I loved, and that didn't require much shoulder movement. It was the plan of action I was about to embark upon.

I began to build my fitness by walking around my local area which contained a lot of hills. I was having a lot of indigestion and would drink Mylanta before and after the walks but it didn't seem to really help. I was struggling to get my fitness back, getting out of breath easily and the indigestion was interrupting my regime.

I went to my diabetic endocrinologist and explained my symptoms and he said it sounded like angina to him, so we had better arrange a stress test. I performed the stress test and at the end, I was asked if I had a cardiologist appointment to go to. When my reply was, 'no,' they told me I had better make one. This was the beginning of a significant journey that would make my type 1 diabetes seem like a walk in the park.

A long story short, I had an angiogram done and three major blockages were found. The aorta was 98 % blocked. It was stented, leaving the other two to be done at a later date because they were in a branch, so were trickier to do. In the Coronary Care Unit (CCU), most of the comments by the nurses were, 'You're a bit young to be here aren't you?'

As a child, I was always told by medical staff that diabetes could lead to blindness and diabetic nephropathy (diabetic kidney disease) which could lead to having some parts of your feet or legs amputated. The heart was never mentioned. Not that it would have made any difference to my attitude towards the diabetes anyway but I just never expected the heart to be a part of diabetic complication.

It was only six weeks after the first stents, from which I didn't seem to get much relief, that I was back in to have the two branches stented. That had a much better outcome and I felt back to normal again.

When I asked the cardiologist how long before I could return to teaching aerobics, he told me he was going to have a job keeping me from having open heart surgery, let alone teaching aerobics. Aerobics was out of the question. Walking and gentle exercise would be the most I could expect. Straight away in my little defiant mind, I thought, 'You're not telling me I'm not going to do aerobics again.' If I set my mind to something, there's no stopping me. 'You just wait and see,' announced the defiant voice. Nothing gets in my way.

After my second lot of stents and slowly regaining my fitness, the Zumba phenomenon was just hitting the workout circuit and Shelley, a girlfriend, told me she had gone to a class and loved it. She took me along with her to a class, which provided another defining moment for me. Hearing that wonderful, rhythmic Latin music, accompanied with Latin moves like Salsa, Mambo and Merengue, just blew me out of the water. This was the perfect combination of rhythm, dance and exercise that would become my next passion.

So, with three stents and the message I would never do aerobics again, I became a Zumba instructor and taught a couple of classes a week. I was addicted to buying all the funky bright trousers, tops and accessories. I loved the bright purple and hot pink cargo pants and mixing the crop tops with a singlet over the top. Bright rubber wrist bands were fun to wear as they coordinated with the outfit beautifully. I even had three pairs of shoes in different colours and styles.

Man, I loved strutting my stuff, looking and feeling great. I had the moves, grooves and clothes to wiggle my hips and pulsate my arms. I was able to do it because it had a wavering effect on the heart rate. Slow tracks followed by a few fast ones ensured the constant climb of the heart rate in aerobics was avoided. It wasn't aerobics but it was more fun and just as beneficial to the body and mind. It was the best thing since sliced bread.

In 2011, Scott was at Lesmurdie High and at the end of that year, I was asked if I was interested in doing some relief work. Initially I said, 'no.' Primary was all I had ever done and I didn't know how I would go with older kids, so they asked me to just do one day and see what it was like. Within one week, I was doing full-time relief work and soon became part of the wonderful team of the Student Services Educational Assistants. I was still able to teach my Zumba classes, they were mainly at night-time. I absolutely loved working at the high school and now I was there with Scott, and Mark would be there the following year. Happy I would be there again for them if they needed me. How perfect was the timing? Thank you, universe.

About six weeks after starting at the high school, I noticed my toe getting sore. Still teaching Zumba but with a lot of pain, I went to the doctor and said I thought I had arthritis in my foot. The doctor looked at my foot and said, 'That's not arthritis. It's infected. I'll give you some antibiotics and come back next week.' I did just that but the pain increased and after a nurse had a probe around in my toe, she announced, 'There's glass in there.' An x-ray was done and sure enough, there were multiple fragments of glass in my toe.

Referred to a toe specialist the next day, I limped into his office and said, 'There's some glass in my toe, can you just dig it out please?' He took one look at my foot and said, 'That's not just glass. Your foot is infected and you need to come into hospital tomorrow morning.'

'Can I come in on Friday as I have relief work planned for tomorrow and can't let them down?'

He said, 'Come in tomorrow night after work then but not Friday.'

A week in hospital, Intra-Venous antibiotics and I was given the diagnosis of osteomyelitis (infection in the bone). I knew what this was because Eddie had it in his hip as a child. The glass had burrowed its way into the bone and infection set in. The glass couldn't be removed for another few weeks because there was too much swelling and the bacterial infection had to be controlled first. A PICC line (peripherally inserted central catheter line), was inserted so IV antibiotics could be delivered directly into my heart and pumped around my system.

Back home, having called my Zumba clients saying I most probably wouldn't be back for a while, I again had restricted movement because of the pain in my foot. A nurse came out each day and changed the bottle of antibiotics.

With Les away, evenings were spent with Scott, Mark and Phoebe, Mark's pet rabbit, sitting on the lounge and watching TV. Phoebe was house trained and had a litter box, so when she needed to go to the toilet she could jump inside the enclosed box with a flap and do her business. She loved hopping up on our laps at night, being cuddled and stroked.

As I sat down on the couch ready to watch TV with the kids, no sooner had Phoebe jumped onto my lap, I bolted up saying in a loud voice, 'Bloody Phoebe has pissed on me, dirty little rabbit,' as I felt this gushing of wetness spread over my lap. As I stood up, Scott shouted, 'Mum, all the stuff in the bottle is spraying out.' Racing out to the kitchen pointing the broken PICC line into the sink, antibiotics under pressure were now shooting out of the end like a mini fire hydrant. Panicked and not knowing what to do, I phoned the hospital. When the ward clerk answered, I told her my rabbit had chewed a hole in my PICC line and what should I do? After a pause, she told me to hold on a minute while she asked someone. Minutes later, back on the line, she said nobody knew what to do and to just wait until the nurse came in the morning to change the bottle of antibiotics. I was concerned as I knew this line went directly into my heart. Could anything bad happen? Apparently not, I guess.

Well, you can imagine the rumours and laughs that were going around in the doctor's rooms once word got around about Phoebe's efforts. When I went into see him the following week, his said, 'So your rabbit chewed your PICC line?' My rabbit experience gave everyone some light relief and I became known ever after as the woman that had the rabbit chew her PICC line.

Six weeks later, the infection specialist put me on oral antibiotics for another three months. I went back into hospital and had the glass removed which meant having my toe debrided to be able to get all the glass out, including all the tiny fragments. When debriding is done, a large part of the area is taken out to remove all the foreign material. Even though the glass was no longer in my toe, the pain of walking around on it was still excruciating and I continuously limped. There was also a lot of nerve pain which I hadn't ever experienced before. Taking a nerve pain reliever made me befuddled and extremely foggy without getting rid of the pain. It was one the worst things I've ever endured.

The end of the year came and being sick and tired of limping, I returned to the foot specialist and told him to just take the toe off. It hadn't healed and I was tired of limping all the time. He agreed but told me before he took the toe off, the circulation in my legs and feet needed to be checked otherwise an amputated toe with no blood supply could turn into an amputated foot.

I went to the vascular surgeon and after having the ultrasounds of the blood vessels in my legs, he noted there was definitely a blockage in the vessel feeding the blood supply to the toes. Another angiogram and stent were performed on my leg, so now that problem was fixed I could go ahead and have my bloody toe removed, finally.

In I went and had my toe taken off. After a few weeks longer than it would normally take to heal, the pain in my foot finally subsided. I never looked back. No pain, I could go back to doing Zumba once more. At first, I was a little self-conscious of wearing open sandals, trying to cover my little nub that was now there instead of my toe. However, after a while I didn't really care, it was now part of me and there was nothing to be ashamed of.

At work just prior to having my toe amputated, Janine decided to throw a morning tea and honour me with a 'Toe-phy'. She used one of her kid's sport trophies, took off the top and mounted a plaster-of-Paris toe on it. Painting the toenail very bright red with a decorative flower on it, the 'Toe-phy' looked very realistic indeed. She topped it off with cup-cakes with toes and finger lollies placed on top.. It was a lovely and fun gesture and that's why I loved working at the school. We were such a close-knit group of colleagues who became very good friends, working and socialising together.

During the remainder of 2012 and up to 2015, I was in and out of hospital at different times having angiograms which usually resulted in having stents. It was becoming part of my normal routine and no one really thought anything of it. I got to know my symptoms, would call my cardiologist directly and would drive myself to the hospital to have the stent done then drive home again.

All this time, I was fluctuating between being able to teach Zumba and feeling pretty good to then getting short of breath. I was using nitrate spray before, during and after any workout to allow the blood to pump more freely around my body, especially my heart.

So, by the time I was 46, I'd had three stents. By 2015, I was going in every four months for a stent. Then my smaller blood vessels were starting to clog up. These, however, were too small to stent and so medication was the only option to help remedy the symptoms. I got to the stage where I couldn't walk up to our local park. I had to give up Zumba and even doing home chores such as vacuuming and making the bed was too hard. There were days when I thought to myself I can't go on like this any longer. I had gone from being an exuberant, fit and energetic person to this slow, pathetic shadow of the person I was before. Friends would have to park close so I wouldn't have to walk far and slow down their pace so I could keep up. I felt like a pitiful excuse of a human being. I never dreamed in a million years, especially in the short space of a few years, that I would have reached this state.

Despite the struggle of an increasingly fragile heart and my inability to do so much, I was fiercely independent about my treatment. Les and the boys knew little of the significance of these trips. That's the way I liked it. Yes, if I were to admit it, my health was a pain in the arse but I only wanted it to be a pain for me, not them. I certainly didn't want the boys to live their lives defined by their mother's bad health and ongoing medical issues. That was part of it. The other part was that amazing resilience in my personality that just keeps coming to the fore when the going gets tough. Not everyone would stomp into the surgeon's office and demand to have their toe off and be pleased when it was.

How Can You Mend a Broken Heart
- Bee Gees

By the time 2015 had come around, I was still having regular angiograms and stents. By this stage, I'd had about 12 stents. That gives you some idea as to how I was travelling, or should I say, how my heart was travelling.

I was maxed out on anti-angina medication and my resting heart rate was 46 bpm's. I was slowed to as low as I could go. I remember when I went to Bali with Hon and then Les and the boys, I had to take floating devices into the pool because I would get too out of breath just trying to keep my head above water.

It was the 4th of August, the day after Mark's 15th birthday, that I had my first visit to a new clinic. My cardiologist had said to me a few months prior there wasn't much more that she could really do for me, all the smaller blood vessels in my heart were blocking up and too small to stent. She suggested sending me to the transplant team to see if they could give me a new heart. It sounded like an easy and simple choice to take. A nice, healthy new heart, what else could be any better? I was in.

I never told anyone except Hon about this adventure I'd decided to embark on; we always shared our secrets. Les and the boys didn't even know; I was protecting them from this escalation in my condition. They didn't need to know unless and until things changed and a heart transplant was definite.

The reason I never wanted to say anything to anyone was quite simple, really. If things didn't work out and I wasn't a suitable candidate, then why worry my hubby and children about it? I have always kept my health issues quite private and never like to make an issue about it. I know there is nothing more boring when people go on about their health issues. Nobody really wants to hear about them and if they say they do, I can guarantee they're just being polite. Let's face it, it's a real party buster and mood-downer when someone starts on about their waning health issues. That's the call for exit stage right, I'm out of here.

When Hon knew I was being referred to the Heart Transplant Clinic, she wanted to come with me to my first appointment. Initially, I told her it was completely fine and I was alright going by myself but as Hon would have it, she insisted on sharing at least the first appointment together. So, to keep Hon happy and I guess it was nice to have someone to share information with, she met me at the coffee shop prior to the appointment. While we were waiting, we were going through some travel magazines as we had planned to go to the west coast of America together in two years-time. We were planning the more rural areas we would like to see so we could start putting money aside to do this together. As you can see, I was always positive about the future, even in the minutes prior to going to my first heart transplant appointment.

So off Hon and I trot to the Fiona Stanley Heart Transplant Clinic, quite excited about the whole prospect of getting my heart swapped out for a new one. Some might say I am naïve. I just say I'm extremely positive and an optimist who takes everything as an opportunity and in her stride.

I remember talking to the new cardiologist on the first day and after going through my history, he asked me, 'So you want a new heart?'

'Yes, I do,' was my simple reply.

'It's not that simple you know,' he replied.

'Yes, it is,' was my easy-going response, with a smile on my face.

'No, it's not,' he stated warily.

Once again I said, 'Yes, it is.' I don't think he quite knew how to take my easy-going attitude.

Part of the cardiac treatment regime was having to go to the cardiac gym. You had to go there two to three times per week where a program of weight resistance and a cardio workout regime is tailored for you. Your heart rhythm, blood pressure and pulse rate are monitored pre- and post- workout. The physio reports back to the clinic each week with a progress report. Hopefully, gains in fitness levels are shown.

Why all the fuss about fitness? There's a fine line in being a transplant recipient; you need to do it while you are relatively healthy so your recovery from surgery will be better. If they perform a transplant when the person is quite ill and not fit, the outcome is severely compromised. With that, I began my trips from school after lunch down to the hospital gym two afternoons a week after lunch.

When I got my next appointment in the mail, I just told Les the cardiologist was sending me to the public sector to see if they had more ideas than her. That resolved the issue of why I was going to Fiona Stanley Hospital.

At the second appointment, I saw the same doctor and he continued with a few more investigations and questions, again telling me it was a long process and there was strict criterion to get on the transplant list. A lot of other things may have to be tried before that point. My response was, 'Well, what are we waiting for? Let's get started with the process, then.' I really didn't see the issue with the whole thing and at the same time, I really don't think the cardiologist understood my very casual and nonchalant approach and positive manner towards it all.

During the third visit, I finally got to meet Dr A, the cardiologist, one of the senior consultants in the team who was to become a central player in my eventual listing for a heart, despite my diabetes. I think he had been filled in on my easy going and positive approach about it all, so he came to find out for himself. We got on really well straight away and it was after this initial meeting with him, things really started to move in a more serious direction.

Dr A told me that when he first received the letter from my cardiologist, he told her it was highly unlikely they would proceed any further with me. I was too much of a high risk, because diabetics usually don't fare well with transplants due to the damaging impact diabetes has on the body's systems. As medical protocol was not to refuse to see any patient, he would at least see me.

All my subsequent visits were with Dr A as he began the investigations of my other bodily and organ functions. He had to make sure my kidneys were alright and able to withstand the drugs needed throughout this process. My lungs and vascular system were scanned and bone density checked. After realising my body was in pretty good shape, he took my case each week to the Thursday meetings. He continued to be told, 'Dr A, stop bringing her to the table. It's not happening, she's too much of a high risk.' Dr A continued believing in me, so I had to get a letter from my diabetes endocrinologist to say that my diabetes was under good control and he thought my body would cope with a transplant.

Next time I went to see Dr A, I must admit reality started to bite when the significance of my condition was revealed to me in plain and simple terms. My endocrinologist specialist had written and said that, given the state of my heart, the next ten years of my life would constitute a slow demise and so a transplant would be the best option. Dr A turned around and said to me, 'I think he's being a little bit optimistic with giving you another ten years.' I asked him, 'Why, how long do you think I have?'

'Five years at the most and that's if your heart doesn't just stop suddenly before that,' came his very direct response.

That hit me like a tonne of bricks. The idea of dying hadn't ever really been in my thoughts. It still seemed it was years before anything would happen, after all, I'd been going along quite happily having stents to keep it going. This could go on forever, couldn't it?

So, driving back to work that morning was the first time it actually hit me. *Five years at the most if not before.* Shit. This was the real thing now. Crying in the car on the way to work, I tried to get myself together. I never cry. The last time I cried was when Beth died. This was a new, overwhelming state for me to be in. My mortality is finite. I had never really thought about not being here with my family. Medics can always find a way to keep you going, can't they?

Arriving at work, I made a coffee and put it out of my mind and the day continued as normal. It had to be normal for my boys. I'm their security and back stop, the strength in their world keeping things normal. With that, I went to class and the day began.

During the October school holidays, I thought I should revamp my bedroom. It had been the same colour and décor for 16 years and if I was going to be some time at home convalescing from a transplant, then I would like to enjoy it in a nice fresh boudoir. Les never suspected anything; I just told him I was sick of the same colour since we had moved into the house and a revamp was well overdue. He was working away, so it didn't really bother him because he wasn't there while I did it. I always loved painting and found the whole process very relaxing as I worked to music and the beautiful wafting aroma of scented wax melts. New carpet, shutters and a change of colour was exactly what the doctor ordered and it was fun buying new bed coverings and accessories. Hon was my interior decorator advisor; she has a natural knack and eye for that sort of thing. I absolutely loved my new personal sanctuary.

A few months later, I could tell another blockage was occurring. Shortness of breath, spraying the nitrate spray regularly, I called my cardiologist and asked her if she would book me in for another angiogram and stent. I had tried going to the emergency department at the hospital as Dr A had told me to do if I got into trouble but after six hours, I went home. I told them, 'I need a stent,' but they said they could admit me to hospital and observe me but they couldn't just give me a stent. Stubbornly, I left and rang my cardiologist and was booked in for following Friday.

This process was so familiar by now, I didn't even bother telling Les I was going for an angiogram. I told Mark and Scott I was going in and if I wasn't home after school, I would be back tomorrow. This was now the 13th heart angiogram, so the boys never even thought anything about it, nor Les for that matter.

Driving myself in, I did the normal routine: greeting all the regular nurses in the cath lab and chatting away while they did all the prep stuff and talking to the cardiologist as well. The insertion through the femoral artery in my leg was proceeding as usual when I heard him on the phone. Something along the lines that he had tried to get it out but couldn't. The balloon he was inserting had broken and it wasn't coming out. He said, 'Colleen, the balloon's broken and I think this may need surgery.'

Again, my casual response was, 'Yep, OK. No problem.' The nurses were now moving quickly around me and I said quite loudly, 'You had better call my husband. He doesn't know that I'm in here today. I drove myself in.'

With what seemed like only minutes apart, the surgeon then appeared while I was still in the cath lab, introducing himself, then the anaesthetist appeared. He asked if I had any problems with anaesthetics before. My reply was, 'no.' I then drifted off thinking that the sweet slumber of the liquid anaesthetic dream state was blissfully being bestowed upon me. I'd actually 'drifted off' into cardiac arrest.

Waking up in intensive care the next day, I was a bit confused about what had happened. I still had a tube through my nose that went down into my stomach. Then I saw Les and Mark arrive. Les told me of the shock he'd had when he received the call saying I was being taken down for emergency open heart surgery, especially without him even knowing I was in here for an angiogram. It was totally a hit way out of leftfield.

Mark was a bit overwhelmed with the tube down my throat and the monitor with a lot of readings was constantly changing rhythms and flashing symbols. Then the nurse told them she was just about to take the tube out. It wouldn't take a minute and they could stay if they wanted to. Being told to take a breath in and then a long breath out, she slowly pulled out the tube on the exhale. That was quite a strange and not particularly pleasant feeling and my body showed its displeasure by throwing up a large volume of green liquid that looked like I had been living in a swamp. Now covered in slimy gump, the look on Mark's poor little face was one of shock and disgust. The nurse quickly told them to hop out while she cleaned me up and changed the bed sheets. Definitely a good move. I thought it was all quite funny but poor Les and Mark, just arriving to see me, were greeted with a scene out of 'The Exorcist' without the 360-degree head turn. You really do have to see the funny side of things, don't you?

The nurse asked me how I felt and I told her that my stomach was really sore, like an elephant had sat on it. She explained that was from all the CPR the girls in the cath lab were doing on me. It took them two hours to stabilize me before they could take me down to theatre. Now it was making sense with the surgeon and the anaesthetist coming in together and me drifting off. I had been going in and out of consciousness while they were resuscitating me with CPR.

Two nurses then popped in and excitedly announced, 'You're awake. We knew you would make it. We just had to come and make sure that you did. We're so glad that everything turned out alright. You really gave us a scare down in the cath lab.' Then as quick as they appeared, they vanished just like that. Happy and reassured that I was still alive and didn't die on the table. Now that made it a bit more real, coming that close to death.

About five days later, I was moved onto a ward and the girls from work came in to see me. It was so lovely to see them. They brought in a gorgeous box of goodies and pressies staff at work had contributed to. Poor Janine felt guilty and was blaming herself for putting me in this state. The day before going in for my angiogram, I'd taught a Zumba class at school in the afternoon. It was part of a fundraiser we were all doing for 'Movember'. I took my nitrate spray before the class, then ten minutes later took another quick squirt to keep the heart vessels dilated to let the blood flow a bit easier. At the end, another recovery spray was absorbed into my mouth and blood stream with much gratitude and relief. That's how I got through still being able to do some of my working out. I reassured Janine that I was already booked in for the angiogram and the Zumba wouldn't have made any difference to having the emergency triple Bypass. I know even to this day she thinks she caused it! You're officially off the hook Janine, it's now in writing!

I was off work for six weeks recovering from the surgery. The worst part, pain-wise from that surgery, was where they took the vein from my leg to do the new plumbing. That took a long time to heal and my leg would blow up like a balloon each day, so I had to keep it elevated whenever I could. I slowly began my fitness recovery by walking up and down our long driveway a couple of times a day. Then up to the end of the street, slowly improving to getting up to our local park and back.

In hospital, the surgeon had told me how he had tried to retrieve the balloon in surgery but even pulling with all his might, it wouldn't budge. That's why he had to bypass all the plumbing and leave the broken balloon in my heart. He went on to say he thought it may be a blessing in disguise as he had rerouted all the vessels that had been stented and he was hoping most of my symptoms would disappear. So, with that, he had taken me off most of my medication for angina, just waiting to see how things go.

I had not long been out of hospital and Scott's best mate, Frank, came around after school to see me. Frank is a very jovial and 'out there' kind of person, with lots of stories and entertaining to be around. When he said to me, 'Mrs Ashby,'–that's what he was used to calling me at school–'you would have to be the unluckiest person I know.'

Absolutely shocked and taken back by this comment, I came back quite quickly and pronounced 'Frank, how can you say that?'

'Well last year you got some glass in your toe and had to finish up getting it amputated and now you go in for a simple angiogram and end up having an emergency triple bypass with open heart surgery. Now, how unlucky is that?' he countered back.

'Yes, but if I never got that glass in my toe and then the infection not healing, I wouldn't have found out I had a blockage in my leg and that could have ended up in a few years' time as a foot amputation. With the broken balloon, well that could turn out to be a blessing in disguise as all my stented arteries have been rerouted. So, you see Frank, both incidents were really blessings in disguise,' I told him pragmatically.

Shaking his head, he didn't know what to think but now at least I made him see the positive long-term blessing to my situation. I truly was shocked anybody would think of me as unlucky. Everything always turns out for me.

Making a good recovery, I was pleased with my progress, except my leg wasn't healing very well and had this disgusting, greenish scabby hole at the bottom. About six weeks later, I noticed that exercise was once more becoming difficult and the angina was kicking in too. Back to the transplant clinic to see Dr A.

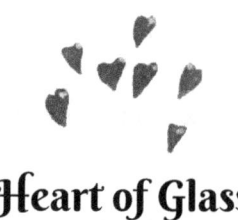

Heart of Glass
– Blondie

Dr A went over the notes of what had happened with the bypass surgery and knowing the symptoms were returning, he booked in another angiogram to see what was going on. Luckily, it was nearly the April school holidays, so I wouldn't have to take any time off work or tell anyone that I was going in. I told Les they were just going to have a look and run some bloods and I would be home again the following day.

Mum dropped me at the hospital, I told the boys I would be home tomorrow and to be good at home for Nanna. I had the angiogram, which revealed one of the new grafts had already completely blocked and a second graft was three-quarters blocked but was below the broken balloon, which they couldn't get past. They were shocked at the extent of blockage and how quickly it had occurred. This was a pivotal point in realising a heart transplant may be the only option.

Dr A came around the next day and told me that we may be going down that track now but there were many more tests to be done. He asked if Les knew about the situation and I told him, 'no.'

'When am I going to meet him?' he asked.

'When you list me. If I don't get listed, he will never know that I have gone down this track. Why would I worry him and the boys about something like this if it doesn't eventuate?' was my answer. With that, I went home and just told the family, 'they're putting me on some new medication to try,' and that was that.

Things were now getting harder to do. I had to drive up to our local park and take Jasper, our little pet dog, for a slow walk. Walking any distance was an issue. Making the bed was now too hard and vacuuming was too demanding. I hated this state of being slowed right down and not being able to do things. Those days of aerobics and Zumba were now like a distant memory, most probably never to be experienced again.

Dr A advised me to go back to my vascular surgeon to look at my leg, perhaps there may be a blockage in the leg that needs stenting but either way, we had to get that sore healed up. He told me if the rest of the team saw my leg, there was no way they would find me suitable for transplant. If I couldn't get my leg to heal, how would I go healing from a transplant? So that was my next challenge.

Back to the vascular surgeon, who booked me in for another angiogram on the other leg and was thinking of debriding my leg, making a new fresh wound to encourage it to heal better. The angiogram was done and the surgeon ballooned part of the blood vessel to open it up a bit more. The following day, he decided not to do anything to my leg in case it made the situation worse. Antibiotics and a wound care plan were the order of the day.

Gradually, my leg did heal and to this day, a red scar any warrior would be proud to wear as a badge of honour is highly visible down my leg. Long skirts and trousers were now a main part of my wardrobe. People may not find a long, red, nasty-looking scar running up the inside of my lower leg very attractive. However, and like my toe, I eventually didn't bother about it. It is part of my personal history and a reminder of all that has kept me alive so far. Now I wear my scars with pride.

By now, I had told Carol at school, it was the only way that I would be able to keep things contained. She told the principal so I would be able to take time off from work for appointments without any questions being asked. Carol was totally understanding and wonderful and I totally trust in her, a truly beautiful and empathetic person indeed.

Quite an amazing coincidence occurred around this time. One of the students at the school, Jaedin, was now going to the same transplant clinic as me. He had been going to the children's hospital with cardiac issues from birth. Now he was older, he had been referred to Fiona Stanley and was also just having to start at the cardiac gym. As Carol knew what I was going through, she thought it may be nice for Jaedin to have someone going through the same health issues to support him, if needed. I knew Jaedin from the previous years and now he was in year 11, we could talk more as adult to adult. I arranged with his parents to take him down to the cardiac gym twice a week. I could introduce him to the staff and people there and he would have some reassurance knowing I was there if he needed me. I was able to give Jaedin's parents some idea of what was in store for him and it gave them both reassurance they had someone they could discuss transplant issues with.

It was now 2016 and I couldn't make it across the school yard to 'J' block or upstairs to maths. Timetables were modified so I could cope physically. My inner circle of trusted friends all knew I didn't like any fuss or too much questioning about my health. I would give information if I needed to. That was the perfect environment for me to be in. 'Business as usual' was the motto I liked to go by.

Aside from the heart thing, family life was cruising along just nicely. Scott was in his final year at school and Mark was into riding his dirt bikes around in the bush in his spare time. He had already built a dirt bike that came in a box of parts from a mechanic workshop, stating that all the parts were there. He was in year 8 when he did this by himself during the Christmas holidays, and without any help. What I thought would take a couple of months, he was riding in six weeks. Motors, engines and anything mechanical, he had a natural knack for. Scott, on the other hand, was a gamer and a wiz on computers and with strategic games. Chalk and cheese but both happy in their own right. All the work focusing on their strengths had paid off.

I just wanted to be around a bit longer to see them grow in to the beautiful, young men I knew they would become. Stephen was ten years older and had been in the workforce for a few years now. He also had a girlfriend and been moving in and out of home, so I knew he was alright out in the big wide world.

Scott and Mark, however, needed a bit more nurturing and guidance in manoeuvring the unfamiliar world beyond school and home life. My job wasn't done yet.

By mid-2016, Dr A decided to admit me to hospital to run some more tests. He also wanted the rest of the team to meet me in person. He had been telling them I was more than just the medical history they've been reading on paper, so this was his chance for the first grand meeting. Once again, I told Les it was just a night or two of running more tests and trying out new meds and with that, I was once again dropped off at the hospital by Mum.

On the second day of being in hospital, the auspicious first meeting was to take place. I was expecting maybe three or four other doctors besides Dr A but, oh no, not on your Nellie. It seemed like a whole rugby team of medics filled the room. Quite overwhelmed, I was sitting perched up in the seated window ledge looking out of the window when I met my audience.

Introductions were done and I met Dr L, Cardiologist, and Clare, Transplant Nurse Practitioner. I can't remember who else was there. Dr L chatted to me, asking me questions and as I relaxed with him, things began to flow easily. He asked me how my family felt about the transplant?

My reply was that they didn't know. I confirmed nobody really knew and, until I was listed, they will never know. Well, with that response from me, the team were all looking at each other, muttering lowly and shaking their heads in their collective agreement that this was not a good idea. I knew it was serious but all I could think of at the time was that they reminded me of a scene out of Monty Python, the one where all the women were dressed as men with fake beards and wanting to participate in the stoning. Women, of course, weren't allowed to participate, so their voices suddenly dropped into a low, deep murmur.

Dr L then took the lead and started out saying that I wouldn't be able to go through something like this without good support. My reply was that I had so far and was coping extremely well. I wouldn't put them through any unnecessary stress until I really had to and again told him, like I had Dr A, unless I was listed, they would never find out I had been down this track. After a bit of bantering and Dr L saying he'd had someone try to do it by themselves before and it didn't work out, they all left the room. 'Exit stage right,' as Snaggle Puss would say.

A couple of weeks after that meeting, Dr A called me say that he had arranged for me to meet Mr R, Surgical Head of the Heart Transplant Service (the Head Honcho). He had done all he could in getting me this far and now it was up to me. I had to sell myself to him. Even though it was a team vote, Mr R had the casting vote. This was to be the make-or-break opportunity; it was all up to me now.

When Mr R did call me in, he shook my hand and introduced himself. My first words were, 'So you're the guy that votes people off the island?'

His quick and jovial comeback was, 'No, I'm more like the grumpy old witchdoctor that hides out in the corner,' and with that, we both relaxed and sat down.

Mr R, of course, ran through all the negative statistics for a 'normal' transplant recipient and then how much greater my risk would be as a diabetic. I would be lucky to make it through the surgery and then, if I do, the first year would be very trying on the body and I would be lucky to make it through. Assuming I did make it, the most they would expect me get out of my new heart would be five years. There are complications that happen within the blood vessels from medication which seem to be worse in type 2 diabetics. With my type 1 diabetes, those complications would be amplified.

When he had run through all those impressive statistics, I simply asked him, 'Well, if all the stats are so bad and negative, then why do you even do them. What about all the successful transplants and why do I have to be one of the negative stats?'

Looking at me after a pause, he said, 'Alright then. Tell me why we should give you a heart transplant?'

Without even hesitating I answered back, 'All right then, if I don't get a new heart, I've most probably got five years at best. Of those five years, it will be a slow demise of not being able to get around or do anything I enjoy and be extremely limited, anyway. If you give me a new heart, even if I only have five years, at least I will be able to be more active, do things with my boys and family, and enjoy them and what's not to say that I make more than five years post-transplant? You give me the heart and I'll look after it.'

With that, he sat back in his chair looking at me and said, 'Fair enough. We'll consider you for transplant.' I walked out feeling I had done a good job on selling myself and Dr A would be proud that all his efforts to this point had paid off. It still had to be taken to the Thursday meeting but I was feeling positive about the outcome. There's certainly nothing like having to sell yourself for a second chance of life, that's for sure.

Dr A phoned me on the Thursday afternoon and told me they would go ahead and list me after a few more investigations had been done. He also told me that now might be the time to tell my husband and the boys. He wanted to meet Les before I was listed.

So now the reality of this whole past year was coming to fruition. It was soon to be game on for real.

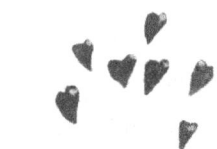

People Get Ready
– Eva Cassidy

Time to tell the family. Friday night after dinner, I decided to tell Les first. Mark was outside doing something in the shed, Scott was in the office on his computer, so I had some quiet time to tell him. I can't remember exactly how the conversation went but I explained how I had been going to Fiona Stanley, well it was really to the Transplant clinic. It had taken a year but they have finally decided to consider me for transplant. Standing at the kitchen sink doing dishes, he stopped and looking at me disbelievingly, questioned back, 'What, a heart transplant?'

'Yes,' was my simple reply.

Taken aback and shocked, Les replied, 'A heart transplant, that's serious stuff. I didn't think you were that bad.'

'Without it, I've most probably got five years, if the heart doesn't just give out suddenly from the strain,' was my explanation. From that point, he asked what I had already been through and why I hadn't told him. I explained the whole scenario with the team and why I hadn't told anyone. Les needed time to process all this, so we sat down on the couch with a cup of tea and put the TV on. I told him I still didn't want anyone else knowing until closer to the time. It was easier than having people asking me how I was every five minutes, have you heard anything yet? And tell me if you need anything done etc. That was just not me and he agreed.

Then Scott popped his little self around into the lounge area and asked, 'So when are you having your transplant, Mum?'

Les and I looked at each other in shock, then back at Scott. 'How do you know about the transplant, Scott?' I asked.

'I heard you and Dad talking in the kitchen. You can easily hear through the wall,' was his innocent reply.

'Yes, I'm going to have a transplant. I still have a couple of tests to do yet and then once I'm listed, it can take anywhere from one week to a year. It's just a waiting game. I'm not telling Mark just yet. I'll wait for the right time, OK darling?' Then with a simple nod of his head, he went back on his computer.

It was a lot for Les to take in. I had no idea just how much Scott would know or be able to comprehend the immensity of having a transplant but the cat was out of the bag now and certainly couldn't be put back in.

Only the following week, Dr A told me he had booked me into hospital for a couple of days while they ran some more tests. On the second day before I was going to leave, Dr A and Clare came around to see me. They both went through the whole process of waiting and then having the transplant, plus post-op care. Then Dr A asked if I had told Les yet? I told him I had and after the initial atomic shock wave, he's all on board.

'Well, when am I going to meet him, then? I'm starting to think he doesn't really exist, he's just a fictitious person,' Dr A half-jovially, half-seriously enquired.

'I can get him in here today if you want?' I told him.

'Now? This afternoon then?' he stated more than asked.

'Sure, I'll call his boss and get him to come over when he gets back to the yard in his truck,' was my agreement.

'OK. Clare and I will come back around 3 pm to meet your mysterious husband,' was Dr A's last words as he and Clare exited the room together.

I called Les's boss and told him that he needed to get to the hospital as soon as he could. Once Les received the message over the truck radio, he returned to the yard and called me before he left. I told him Dr A wanted to see him this afternoon before I can leave. 'They want to talk to you in person.' With that, Les was on his way.

Les came in my room in his work clothes and I reassured him it didn't matter that he was in those clothes. Then Dr A and Clare returned at 3 pm as promised. The welcome was warm with laughs and smiles and a few jokes about how they thought he was just a figment of my imagination. They went on to explain the situation a lot better than I had and with more medical detail, to reassure Les but also let him know it wouldn't be an easy road ahead. Now they had finally met my very real husband, that box had now been ticked, thank God.

I was now able to tell the very few close friends who knew about the transplant that it was now happening. It made it a little easier being able to share some of this information, it was not only intriguing and new for me but even more so for them. Let's face it, how many people know someone who has been through a heart transplant before? Certainly not me, that's for sure. To all the friends with whom I confided at that time, thank you all for your trust, support and secrecy on my behalf.

One of the things everyone gets told to do before getting listed is to get their affairs in order and try and take out a life insurance policy. Well, I filled out the form for the life insurance policy and as you can guess, after filling out previous health history, they came back saying, sorry but you are not suitable to have this policy granted. No surprise really, was it Batman? At least I could update my will, which I was able to do online.

Then I thought I had better arrange my funeral. I wrote a letter from me to my loved ones and family, along with the music and procedure for the funeral. I didn't want a sad funeral, after all, it's about celebrating the life of the person and I am a very positive, bubbly and fun kind of person. Sad and melancholy is definitely not my style. I even stipulated that, instead of rosemary being placed on the coffin by mourners, I wanted lollies. Liquorice All Sorts, Turkish Delight and some assorted lollies to choose from and to eat on the way to the coffin before saying goodbye to me. Now that is the perfect send off for a type 1 diabetic, don't you reckon? My songs were all upbeat and I would want people to chat about their memories of me in a joyous and happy way, no crying, you can do that later if you really feel like you need to but not on my shift, baby.

I was busily typing away at my desk having a bit of a break when Carol walked in to check on me and see how I was going. When I turned around and told her I was just typing my funeral plan, she quickly turned around and said, 'Oh, I'll leave you to it then,' and hot-tailed it out of there. Funny seeing how people react when you're openly entertaining the idea of your finality. Mortality is something people really don't like to think about or entertain. I was quite enjoying imagining being at my funeral, listening to uplifting music and wondering which lollies would I choose if I had to pick one? Hmmm... Liquorice All Sorts or Turkish Delight? I think I would just have to take both.

One of the tests prior to transplant surgery is to check for antibody levels. The higher the antibodies in the blood stream the greater the risk of rejection with the new donor tissue. Females always have a higher count than men if they have had children. With each pregnancy, new antibodies are produced. I may have three children but I've had five pregnancies, which meant my antibody levels were high. As it turned out, my antibodies were nearly all of what they call high level ones, which meant issues with rejection were a real concern. With that in mind, the last test was another breast screen to make sure there were no signs whatsoever of cancer. Having that last box ticked, I was now officially listed for transplant. It took exactly one year to get to the point of being a suitable candidate for a new heart. A sigh of relief as the round one battle had been won. The bell had been rung and the clang rang out loud and clear. Hallelujah!

Life went on around me in the secret bubble. Sometimes I had to be quick in my thinking to not let anything slip out accidently in conversation. It was certainly a relief not having to explain or talk to people all the time about my health. I could always just breeze over the subject quite vaguely then change it. I was a master of being able to do that.

Scott was getting excited as he only had a few weeks of school before graduation. Mark was looking forward to being in the class that Scott had been in that year. Plus, I had just found out Stephen had gone into a long-term rehab centre. That was a big relief for me, knowing what he had been going through over these past few years with his addiction. I truly hoped this would be a turning point for him in his life. I love him deeply and hate to see his life moving in this downward spiral. He has such a beautiful and loving heart and is a kind person. Unfortunately, drugs and alcohol have destructively taken him to a darker side of being. My hope and love are with him always.

A quiet 52nd birthday was celebrated. Scott had now finished school and Mark was enjoying the September school holidays. He had obtained his learner's permit at the beginning of the month and was extremely happy he could drive everywhere. Mark had been driving to school with me, to the shops and any excuse for an opportunity to get behind the wheel. Les and I had told Mark about the transplant and a bit like Scott, it was hard to judge his reaction but at least he was now in the inner circle of knowing. One thing with my boys, they would never say anything to anyone, that's for sure.

Once we had told Mark, Clare told me to bring in both boys along with Les and she would explain about the transplant in an easy way for them to understand. She also said she could show them where the ICU was so it would be familiar to them. We did exactly that and Clare did a great job with explaining and drawing simplified diagrams on a whiteboard about how the antibodies attack a foreign body in the system and how the anti-rejection drugs work to avoid this. Stick figures of sheep and grass with three fences at increasing heights were used to resemble the process. Even Les and I gained a much better understanding of what the different drugs do, which is important when you're swallowing all these tablets every day, twice a day.

The one thing about the transplant clinic is it's a very friendly and family-like unit. Doctors, nurses and anyone else working there are all called by their first name. Casual chats and laughs are a definite must, home baked goods are happily accepted, too. Close bonds and trust are forged here, especially since you are connected to this extraordinary unit for the rest of your life. Personal connections are made over the huge amount of invested time in each person.

Most of us who have been transplanted eventually get to know one another and share a common bond. It truly is a unique and exceptional unit.

I still had to go to the cardiac gym and on one of these visits, I ran into Dr A walking through the hospital. He told me they had already found a suitable donor heart but when they put my blood in with the donor tissue, I just destroyed it in the test tube. The high antibodies had already revealed their destructive power on attacking any incoming invaders. Dr A asked if Les could give a blood sample so they could find out exactly where the strong antibody was coming from to try and isolate it. If it wasn't him, they needed a blood sample from Paul, my first husband, if possible.

Les gave the blood sample and with any antibody testing it takes a bit of time to do due to the complexity of the process. About the same time as the results were coming through another match was found and again, like the previous test of compatibility, I won over and destroyed the donor tissue. My antibodies were triumphing in battling the invading tissue. This, however, was a time where I wished I could let this fight go and not rule so victoriously.

The team had now isolated the 'Mike Tyson' on my antibodies and yes, it came from Les. Les, I always knew you were strong. Anyway, now they knew exactly what antibody to try and match against, the screening process could be refined. Due to the two previous very negative results, Dr A said the team had come up with a new plan to give me a higher probability of a successful match without rejection.

He told me they will often do this procedure post-transplant if the patient keeps on going into rejection. As my antibodies were being quite an issue, they wanted me to do it pre-transplant. I had to have my entire lymphatic system radiated. Radiating my lymph nodes would stop the production of antibodies for a while. This way, when a suitable heart was found, my antibodies would be much lower, meaning a larger chance of success. That was the plan.

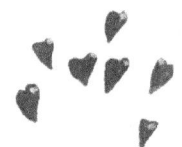

Get Ready for This
– 2 Unlimited

It was now term 4 in the school year and my first appointment at the cancer radiation centre was to tattoo the lymph nodes and then make a full body mould, which I would wear during radiation to keep me in position and as still as possible. A warm, pliable mesh plastic is gently placed over your whole body, including your head. You can still breathe as the mesh holes are quite large but it still makes you feel a bit claustrophobic. It sets quickly and then the mould is lifted off and hung up in the racks with your name and number on it. It was interesting to see how they perform radiation treatments and the detail involved. Now I was prepared to begin the treatments.

I drove myself, as always, down to the radiation centre and waited for my name to be called. When it was, the nurse took my full body mould from a rotating rack used for storing all the moulds. Lying on my bed, my body was lined up with the tattoos, then the mesh body mould was placed and locked down. Told to take deep breaths, the procedure began with me alone in the room. Now, I'm pretty good with this sort of stuff but when you're locked down tight in this sarcophagus-like contraption, it makes your mind go into a stress state. Low level panic began to rise, so I reminded myself to keep breathing. In no time, it was over and the claustrophobic sarcophagus was removed. I had six treatments a few days apart, over two weeks. Another box was now ticked. It really wasn't that bad but it's strange how your mind can just take over and you lose a little bit of sanity for a few fleeting moments.

Apart from getting a little tired, I managed to keep going to work without too much trouble. Then Dr A called to tell me they now wanted me to have two weeks of plasmapheresis. Now that my body would stop making any new antibodies, he wanted to try and wash away the old ones in my system. The appointments were every second day spread over two weeks, so with that, I arranged with Carol to get off early to go to these appointments. There was only two weeks of school left until the end of the school year, so things were slowing down. The girls at work just thought I was going to doctor's appointments, otherwise it went unnoticed.

It was interesting to see how plasmapheresis (a process in which plasma–the liquid part of the blood–is separated from the blood cells) treatment works. You are hooked up to a machine that takes the plasma out of your blood and empties it into a collection bag. The machine then replaces your plasma with new plasma. The whole process takes about an hour and a half. The treatment did make me tired. Thankfully, it was nearing the end of the school year.

I had two more treatments and was booked in for the last two when Dr A called asking me not to bother with the rest of the treatments. When I asked why not, he confirmed the treatments hadn't worked in lowering my antibody levels, so it wasn't worth continuing with any further treatments. A bit disheartened that the treatment hadn't worked, I could now be home for the Christmas holidays and hope that I receive my new heart over this time. My plan was to finish getting the house freshened up a bit.

Scott had finished school eight weeks previously and had been enjoying his time at home gaming and chilling for a while but like all good things, it had to come to an end. I told him that finding a job was now his priority and with a bit of help from an agency, he was soon employed at a car yard. Starting off with washing cars was fine for someone who hadn't had any prior employment experience. Scott was officially in the workforce now, earning money and participating in keeping the country running. I was relieved and happy he at least got a job.

Before Christmas, I had one more appointment at the transplant clinic. With the assurance I'd have my bag packed and phone with me at all times just in case, I left the clinic and drove home hoping for a new heart as soon as possible.

After sharing a wonderful fun-filled Christmas by the pool with friends, life went on a usual, with Mark busy mucking around with his dirt bikes in the shed and looking for any excuse to get in some driving practice to make up his hours towards his licence.

New flooring was ordered for the house and I was getting excited about freshening it up and having it ready for when I got my transplant. Les had been painting the doors and frames during his couple of weeks off over Christmas, so it was like a busy beehive preparing the house for the big event.

New Year was a quiet one, we never did much at this time except for the turn of the millennium. Who remembers all the hype and scare over the turn of the calendar for the year or so before 2000 ticked over? The world was worried that all the computers would crash and the destruction of business's, banks, people's bank accounts and financial institutions would be compromised. Yes, the year 2000 was definitely going to be a turn of a century that we would all remember. Well, what a fizzle it turned out to be. It was, however, a good reason to have a New Year's party, so we did just that. Scott was only one-year old and I had just found out I was pregnant with Mark. That was a good enough reason for celebrating if nothing else.

2017 arrived, quite uneventful but pleasant all the same. We had told Mum about the transplant but I told her I still wasn't letting anyone else know. It could still be months before I got a heart and I preferred to keep it quiet. Mum was pleased but shocked at the same time and had to go through the same mind processing we all did. I never told her I had to have the radiation or the plasmapheresis treatment, I figured learning about the transplant was enough to think about. Les went back to work and I was planning on catching up with a couple of friends from work, which was the norm for that time of year. I remember talking to the few girls at work that knew about how excited I was. With a new heart, I would be able to go back to doing some 'step classes' and aerobics once again.

It's interesting how long it takes me sometimes to come to terms with some of the developments in my life. Take my Zumba classes, for example. It was sometime after I was going to the transplant clinic, with the prospect of getting listed not looking great and my health deteriorating quite dramatically, that I came to the realisation I couldn't ever see myself getting back to being able to participate or teach Zumba ever again. It took me until that time to get rid of all my gear (keeping only one outfit because I couldn't bring myself to completely close that door). That was really emotional for me. Zumba was my passion and joy; it was like part of me had died.

Reflecting on it, I'm seeing my character come to the fore in this example. It took until I could hardly walk to realise I probably wouldn't do Zumba again. I don't think it's someone daft coming to this realisation but someone supremely positive and confident in her own capacity to survive and thrive. As I've mentioned before, I'm not sure why I'm like this but I am and I'm comfortable in my skin with the confidence and positivity it brings me. That doesn't mean I don't get pissed off when life throws me lemons. I do.

I eventually bring myself round to make lemonade. It's just so much easier to be positive than pissed off.

Throughout this time, I was seeing an amazing Bowen therapist. When I came across Tracy, I immediately loved the way she worked and her beautiful spiritual nature. I connected with her straight away and after a session, revealed my secret about the transplant. When I saw her just before Christmas, for some reason the vibe was different. Tracy told me she thought my new heart would be coming in the next three weeks, it was just her gut-feeling. Excited about this premonition, it lifted my energy and confirmation that what I had been visualising was in the same alignment. I felt the benefits of the Bowen as my muscles and body loosened and re-aligned.

Part Three

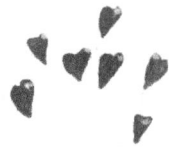

Total Eclipse of the Heart
– Bonnie Tyler

January 2017, just five months after being listed for the transplant and halfway through the school holidays. I had arranged to meet two friends from work to have lunch after my normal clinic appointment at the hospital. I put on my pretty navy-blue summer dress and makeup and off I drove to the hospital for my 8.30 am appointment. I was feeling quite excited because the new flooring was being installed the next day and I was also looking forward to catching up with my friends.

I parked the car and walked up to the clinic and waited to be called in. When I was called in by Dr A, he asked how my Christmas had gone and how was I doing? We had a friendly chat catching up over the past few weeks. I told him I was meeting friends for lunch and about the flooring going in the next day. Then he asked me if I was still wanting the heart transplant?

I said, 'Of course.'

'Well we've got a perfect match,' he said.

'Great,' I replied with excitement.

'But it's happening today,' was his reply.

I looked at him in shock.

In a more assertive voice he said, 'Right now.'

'Should I phone Les and tell him?'

'It might be a good idea,' he replied.

So, I phoned Les and left a message with his boss to tell him to meet me at the hospital as soon as possible because the heart transplant was happening today. Then I rang my friend Dee and told her I wouldn't be able to make lunch as I was getting my new heart. The new flooring was going in tomorrow and if Les was at the hospital, would she be able to be there when the men came to install? Dee confirmed she'd sort out the flooring guys but was just as flabbergasted as I was. Dr A just sat there while I made my phone calls. Apparently, I also called Hon and said I would see her in the morning when I woke up in the ICU. She told me later I sounded like I was just going in to get my tonsils out.

I don't remember anything from making the two phone calls to Les and Dee. I don't even remember Les and Mark coming while I was getting ready for the surgery. Les told me later the last thing I said as I was getting wheeled down on my bed to the surgery was not to forget to feed Jasper, our dog. Les was told to go home as the surgery would go into the night and he could come back in the morning. They would give him a call when the surgery was over.

After the transplant, the family were told the operation had not gone well and to expect the worst. As a rule of thumb, the maximum time allowed on life support with your chest open waiting for the new heart to start is two days. I was on life support for four days before my new heart started to beat independently, albeit tentatively.

During those days, I lived a parallel existence, through the prism of a very, very bad dream. A nightmare of incredible proportions. I cannot stress how bad this dream was or the impact it had on me for many, many months after the transplant. This dream was central to me having post-traumatic stress disorder (PTSD), which manifested sometime after the transplant and for which I needed to eventually seek help.

As part of my therapy for PTSD, I wrote a transcript of this hellish dream. Writing down what I dreamed whilst in an induced coma, effectively hovering between life and death, helped me confront this nightmare and put it away for good.

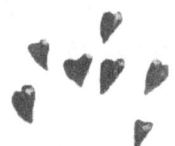

Welcome to My Nightmare
– Alice Cooper

I have struggled with the full transcript of my nightmare being part of my book or not. It was what I experienced for four days while in an induced coma and once I came out of the coma, my mind struggled with reality for a long time. I spent many hours reliving it in all its awful and depressing detail, trying to make sense of it all. My psychologist, Jacqui, told me I may never be able to make sense of it and it was my brain's way of giving a 'reality' to the senses of sound and touch I still had while in the coma. For whatever reason, I still somehow have a bizarre attachment to it and I want to share it with you.

I do not expect you to get it. It's nonsensical and just plain strange. It's dark most of the way through. In the dream, I am overwhelmed by a conspiracy of which I know nothing but am being blamed. Movies and books from my childhood make an appearance. Why? Who knows? It's what my brain threw up when I was so vitally compromised and at death's door.

It is a Saturday in January and I am at my son Scott's best friend Frank's 21st birthday. The party is well under way with all of Frank's family and friends. As most 21st celebrations go, there is music, *drinking and food, a great time being had by all. Scott comes to me and tells me he and Frank want to go and try some marijuana and there was a well-known Indian chief in his tee pee who has good quality stuff. I tell them I will go with them to make sure they are safe and stay while they try it. So off we go across some fields until we arrive at the tee pee. The Indian chief welcomes us all and invites the boys inside. He asks me if I want to come in too but I tell him no, I will sit outside and wait for the boys to finish. The Indian chief follows me outside and gives me a peace pipe, telling me to have a smoke of it as it will help pass the time, he would look after the boys. I take the pipe and pull a long drag on it. The Indian chief goes back inside the tee pee. I sit on the green grass looking out on this beautiful still summer's night, amazed how bright and shining the stars are.*

The next thing I know, the boys have come out and, seeing me collapsed on the grass, pick me up carry me down the hill, then come across a river they need to cross to get to the hospital. As I come in and out of consciousness, I'm aware of the struggle they are both having to lift my limp body up over their heads as they wade through the water chest deep. They finally make their way to the other side of the riverbank and see the hospital entrance close by.

As they hurriedly carry me to the emergency department, the doctors come running out to find out what's happened. The boys tell them they just found me collapsed and bought me here. The doctors tell the boys I am in a diabetic coma from low blood sugar and chastise the boys, saying that any longer and I would be dead; how could they be so irresponsible? Scott tells them I was listed for a heart transplant and they have to help me.

The doctors tell the boys to go home and that they will take care of me. They take me into a cubicle and give me some glucose to raise my blood sugar level and then begin to question me. As they start to unpack my story about how I got into that state, I tell them about the boys trying some marijuana. I admit I had a puff of the peace pipe while I waited for them. Then follows an interrogation, with the doctor's making out I am really a drug user and I won't be getting the heart transplant. As they stand around condemning me, I try to explain that I'm not a drug user and it was a one-off thing; I never use it and I was just making sure the boys were safe. I feel so powerless and unjustified, they won't listen to me at all. I plead with them that it isn't true and that I need the transplant or I will die. It isn't fair.

I am back in the heart transplant clinic talking to the head of the team asking when will I be getting my new heart? He replies in a sinister voice, 'You won't be getting a heart; nobody will be getting a new heart. This whole idea of taking someone's organs and giving them to another person is outrageous and wrong. Haven't you noticed that anyone who has been transplanted has died? We make out they died on the table or of complications afterwards but we only let a few survive so we don't get found out.' I sit there in disbelief, not knowing what to think.

'No,' I say, 'that can't be true. I don't believe you. How can this really be happening after all the clinic appointments and people that have been transplanted?'

'All of us here in the clinic are on the same team not wanting any transplants to be successful, so eventually they will see no point in trying to save lives this way. We will win, you just wait and see,' he answers.

Sitting there in a state of total disbelief, I plead, 'What about Jaedin? He is only young and needs the transplant. He is a beautiful boy and deserves to live a longer life.'

'If Jaedin goes ahead with the surgery, then we will make sure he has no anaesthetic and he will feel every part of the surgery and

will die anyway. We will make sure of it,' he responds with such conviction in his voice.

'But what about me? I have my two boys at home, Mark is still in high school and Scott has only just graduated. They both still need me; I want to see them grow up a bit longer and see them grow into young men.' I say, defeated.

'We wouldn't give you a new heart anyway, you're too old and ugly. If we did decide to give you a heart then this would be your choice, you can have the heart transplant and watch your boys grow up for the next six months but then we will have both of your sons killed without anyone knowing, or you can go without the transplant and see how long you have with them before you die,' he says in a matter-of-fact tone.

'But that's not fair. I don't want them to die because I get to live. I also want to see them grow up,' I state in a disheartened but also vexed manner.

There I am, thinking about all the doctor has told me. I think about how unfair it is for Jaedin and what he will have to go through and there is nothing I can do about it. I can't tell him. The doctor said I would be killed if I tried. I don't want the boys to die and I want to see them grow up a little longer. I am in a state of hopelessness and despair.

Next thing, I am driving down a country road, in a forested area somewhere near Busselton to where the hospital had been moved. I have a strange feeling about it but this is where the transplants are being done now, or so I had been told by the doctors. I park the car in the eerily empty car park and go inside the huge building. I am greeted there by all the normal clinic staff, so feel a bit more relaxed about the strange situation.

They walk with me down the corridors to the private rooms, which are very large and high and have a very weird feel about them all. Dr A reassures me about the whole procedure; I will be taken care of very well. I trust him, he was the one that fought my case for 12 months in clinic to get me listed for the transplant.

He shows me into my room and I meet the nurse that will be looking after me. She has a strong South African accent and is quite tall with auburn coloured hair. She is very jovial and welcoming, which makes me feel a bit more relieved. Dr A says goodbye and leaves the room. The nurse gets me settled and changed into a hospital gown. I sit there on the bed looking around this huge, cold, dimly lit room with tall grey walls and a nurse's desk near the door.

The next thing I remember is waking up back in my room. The nurse is doing my obs, saying the transplant had been done but it wasn't the right heart. I am trying to work out what is going on, nothing is making sense. The nurse tells me not to worry and she will take care of me until a new heart was ready.

It is night-time and she comes to give me some sedatives to help me get a good night's sleep. I take the tablets, swallow them with a glass of water, then settle down for a much-needed rest from this insane situation I was in. Perhaps in the morning things might seem a little better.

My dreams take me into this strange place where I am a boy walking through a jungle filled with all sorts of animals and plants. I am like Mowgli, the Jungle Book boy and have no fear of this place. Snakes and pythons slither through the branches of the tall trees with green vines hanging from them. The colours are amazing, bright reds, pinks and orange flowers scattered throughout this beautiful jungle. A black panther strides by and glances at me without much regard. I can climb the tall trees and swing from the vines, feeling totally free and easy. I can't believe how many huge pythons are all around me, like I am one of them.

When I wake up in the morning, the nurse asks me how I slept? I don't tell her about the dream but just say I slept well. The day *seems to drag without much happening. Night comes around again and I am given the same tablets to help me sleep. I enter the same dream space that I was in the night before, only this time, it is like my room is filled with the jungle painted all over the walls but alive with movement. It is all around me as if keeping me company in this place and once again, I feel completely safe and comforted by the pythons and snakes slithering through the jungle vines and branches. My room is filled with vibrant colour and movement.*

The next morning, I ask the nurse if I can go for a bit of a walk around the corridors to get out of the room for a while. She takes me by the hand as I get out of the bed and as we start to walk, I feel the cold floor beneath my bare feet. As we walk past the rooms I hear the moaning and cries coming out of the doors. It makes me very anxious and worried about what is ahead of me, like being trapped in a prison with no phone call to make and no one coming to visit me, either.

When we return to my room, the nurse tells me I won't be getting my proper heart anymore. Shocked, I ask her why not?

In a venomous voice, she tells me the dreams I had been having over the past few nights are because I am part of the conspiracy movement. She tells me if I wasn't, then I would be having dreams of being a female and no snakes would be there. When I ask her how she knew about the dreams, she tells me the drugs I was given let them see my dreams on the monitor. I am told I will be held there indefinitely and tortured until I tell them all about the conspiracy group and where the headquarters are. When I plead with her that I'm not part of this whole conspiracy thing, she just laughs and walks out of the room, locking the door behind her.

The surgeon and the team come running down the corridors, which are now jiggered rock-lined tunnels glowing with red and black light, just as you might see in a movie depicting an underground tunnel leading to hell. They come bursting into my room saying in a hurried and flustered manner they had the right heart for me this time and they needed to take me straight away to surgery to do the second transplant. They are darting around the room getting things ready as I just sit there in bed watching this circus of medical staff buzzing around me. Then, as I am being hurriedly wheeled out of the room and down these scary hell-bound corridors, the surgeon tells me in a jovial manner that it's going to be successful this time. With these words and seeing the smile on his face, I finally feel like things are going to be alright.

Next, I am recovering from the second surgery and the South African nurse is still looking after me and seems to be quite caring, with a kinder pitch to her voice. I am in a different part of the hospital where all the rooms are in a row but out in the open. There is grass outside and a covered walkway that runs along the extensive passageway. The day is bright and sunny with a sense of calm. Clare, the transplant nurse, comes to see how I am going and to tell me she will be sharing the nursing with the South African nurse. I feel quite OK about this, seeing her petite frame and blonde hair. Clare says she will be up at the main nurse's station if I need anything. I notice that the whole time she is in the room she is holding a mobile phone in her hand, which is a little unusual for a professional person to do.

As I lay there in bed, I call out for Clare to come and help me. After yelling out for what seemed like hours, the South African nurse comes in to see what I need. I tell her I want to talk to Clare but she hasn't come. The nurse tells me Clare is having some problems, she isn't coping well and is spending all her time on the phone trying to sort out her issues. The nurse doesn't think I will get much response from her at all while all this is going on. Even though what is going on in Clare's life shouldn't interrupts her work life, I feel the nurse shouldn't be telling me things about Clare's personal life, either. A duality of emotions bubble around inside me, abandonment by Clare and betrayal by the nurse.

The next day, there is commotion going on and we all need to be moved out because of some emergency. I can see all the other patients being moved out, some are being walked out and others in wheelchairs, then finally the beds are being moved out along the passageway. The South African nurse is just sitting there in her chair doing nothing when I finally yell at her to go and get Clare or at least some help to move me out. She walks out of the room saying she would go and find some help. I am left lying there all alone, feeling very angry that the nurse wasn't doing her job properly. How could she just sit there ignoring me and everything that was going on around us all? Too goddam lazy and self-absorbed. I am filled with fury.

Eventually, the nurse comes back with two men, one tall and muscular and the other much smaller and slightly built. I said to the nurse, 'How are they going to move me? They're not hospital workers and don't know the protocol. They won't know how to manoeuvre the bed or where to go.'

'Don't you worry about it we'll take care of it all. You just lay there and let us do the job.'

The tall man goes off to the storeroom, returning with a roller trolley to put the bed on as it didn't have wheels. After some jolting around and me feeling like I was going to topple out of bed, we are all off and rolling along quite smoothly.

Before I know it, I am being interviewed by a woman in the conspiracy sector. She is insisting that the sooner I realised I was part of this movement, things would get easier for me. I once again, in a very exhausted manner, reply that I am not part of it and never would be.

She replies, 'Don't you realise you are the Queen of this setup? You are the centrefold girl of all the porno magazines, all the girls look up to you and want to be in your situation. You have met all the top Hollywood movie stars and are the celebrity at all the best parties. Men just adore you, you have the most amazing wardrobe, mink coats, high heels and expensive diamond earrings you wear without any regard to the cost of it all?'

I sit there in total bewilderment. How can this be true? I couldn't remember anything of what she had told me and I couldn't believe I would ever be part of anything like that. It just isn't me.

The woman takes out computer, retrieves some archived files and opens them up. As I watch, I see myself being filmed for some porn movies and then film segments at huge parties with hundreds of stars with me at the centre. I can't believe it. But there I was, in full colour picture. But how? I watched myself being so confident and flaunting my power with my gorgeous body adorned in the most glamorous and slinky clothes. It had to be true. Why can't I recollect any part of these memories she was showing me? It had to be fake, made up to convince me to become part of the conspiracy.

'You know your best friend Dee? Well she is your understudy. She has been watching and following everything you do, hoping that one day she would be able to take your crown and become queen herself. If you don't remember all of this part of yourself, you will lose it all. Money, fame, power but most of all being head of the conspiracy.' The woman states in a forceful manner.

'I don't believe you. Dee wouldn't be part of this either, I know her too well. She is like me in her beliefs and standards,' I respond with gumption.

'You have no idea who is part of this conspiracy. We are working on getting the whole world under our control so we can rule with world domination. We have ways of filtering through everything. The coffee you use at work has the drug infused in it and nobody knows or can tell it's in there. The sweetener packs have got it in them and soon we will be able to put it into the water. Then we will have world domination.'

Thinking back to all the girls at work, making coffee and how some of them used the sweetener, I begin to wonder if they are all under its control. No. Surely not. How many then at school were part of this and I didn't know?

As she sits there watching me inwardly question it all, she states, 'John, your Principal and Carol are both right up there in the higher ranks of this all. Most of the teaching staff are already in it too, along with nearly all the Education Assistants. You need to come on board too. You just have to remember or if you can't, then just sign up anyway. It's inevitable, you can't do anything by yourself. You don't have enough power to do so.'

I am sitting there in a totally alien head space, unable to comprehend all this information I had been given. What do I believe?

Waiting in suspense wondering what will happen next, I am sitting on a wooden chair in the middle of a huge, bare room, all white with no windows. The door opens and in walks the woman who was trying to convince me to be part of the conspiracy. She states in a very calm and calculating voice, 'We have got both your boys and your husband, Les. We have all of them tied up and they will all be dead in 24 hours if you don't come over to the conspiracy side. We also have your dog Jasper. Oh, don't worry, we won't kill him as we don't believe in killing animals. We will keep him and slowly torture him by pulling out his teeth one by one and not feed him.'

Tears stream down my face as I think about my beautiful boys and loving husband being killed and what they must be going through all because of me. My poor darling Jasper, so little and innocent he doesn't deserve to have that happen to him. What is the point of having the heart transplant if everything I cared about was gone? I am beside myself.

'But why? My boys are young and innocent and have nothing to

do with this and Les is just a good, loving husband who loves me and the boys so much. Keep them out of this.' I answer back.

'No, you have the power to change it by coming over to our side. You can't win. Those that don't join will be exterminated, we have the power,' she replies.

I knew this whole conspiracy thing was evil and I had to stand against it but I couldn't let my family die. I felt so hopeless and alone.

I have been moved to another room in a separate stand-alone building. The room is more like a huge hall that has the door on a higher level with a short walkway leading to a stairway that lands on the floor I am on. I am quite sick at this stage, not feeling very well at all. The doctors have to put me on plasmapheresis to try and wash some of my antibodies out of my blood as they are too high and starting to attack the new heart. I know what this process is as I had to have two weeks of this treatment before the transplant to try and lower my antibody level. I would just have to lie there while the machine took the plasma out of my blood and then put new plasma in.

A new nurse has come in to change shift and as the nurse that had been looking after me gives her the handover, I notice her ask the new nurse if she has worked with this machine before? The new nurse says that even though she is an agency nurse, she is quite familiar with it all. As I lay there listening and watching the nurses converse, I have a bad feeling about her. Something just doesn't feel right.

The regular nurse finishes the handover and then walks up the stairs and leaves my room. The new nurse comes towards me and says she will be looking after me for the next few hours and that I will soon be feeling much better. The room is uncomfortably warm and the air still and stuffy. I am watching the nurse handle the bag of plasma and start changing the control and buttons on the machine. I know this isn't normal and none of the other nurses had changed anything on the machine before. She gives me a sideways glance to see if I was noticing what she was doing. I quickly divert my glance, staring straight ahead of me, hoping she hasn't seen me looking. I start to panic and am madly trying to work out how I am going to get another nurse to come in and help as I knew something wasn't right.

The nurse pulls out a blue notepad from her white uniform pocket and starts to write something down. She occasionally glances over towards me then continues jotting her notes. She doesn't seem to change her manner or body language. Was I just making all this up in my head? I begin to feel bad that I had thought of her in this negative manner when she may be a very kind and lovely person and not this sinister monster I was imagining her to be. She then just sits back in the chair watching the plasma machine do its work, saying it will be all over soon and I won't be a problem anymore.

Panic grips my whole being once more. What could I do, lying here in this bed and no way of getting any help? I knew then she was also part of this conspiracy and had been sent to kill me. Our eyes meet and we just stare at each other for what seems like an eternity. Her eyes bear the look of sheer contempt and victory.

Just then, the door opens and in walks the nurse who had been looking after me previously. As she strides down the steps, the conspiracy nurse looks at me in a quiet state of defeat, knowing she was soon to be found out. The nurse arrives at my bedside and is looking over at the controls on the machine and then asks the nurse what had she done? The nurse tries to weasel her way out of it by saying the machine was playing up, so she was trying to rectify it. The nurse can see the terror in my eyes as I am looking at her. She then tells the other to get out and never come back again.

After the nurse changes the controls back and puts in a new bag of plasma, she tells me that I will be OK in no time at all. She smiles *kindly at me and tells me she will stay with me until she can find a regular nurse to take over. I wondered if she knew the nurse was of a malevolent intent. All I knew was at that very moment, I was safe and there were obviously people that weren't part of this conspiracy.*

There is a huge gathering of people on the oval in front of the hospital room I am now in. It is like a commentator's box with large windowpanes overlooking the grassed area. Clare, Dr A and Dr L are all in my room conferring about what has to be done next, my health is deteriorating quickly. They come to the same conclusion that I need to be on dialysis, my kidneys were failing and it had to happen now.

Outside, the large group of people are all enjoying the beautiful sunny day, music playing, children running around having fun and the crowd are all drinking from fine wine and champagne glasses while catering staff, dressed in white shirts and black pants and skirts, pass tapas around on fine silver trays. I lay there hazily watching the whole scene wondering what it is all in aid of.

Slowly, a small man enters the crowd unseen by everyone, they are too deep in their own merriment and conversation to notice him. As I watch from my bed in a very drowsy state, I notice he is carrying a semi-automatic weapon across his back. He is quite short, wearing brown trousers and a brown knit jumper with lace-up leather shoes. He has short brown hair and seems to be quite well-kempt.

It was then like a scene unfolding in slow motion as the man pulls his weapon up over his head and is holding it in front of his body. People start to notice him and the screams begin as panic starts to filter through the crowd. He then lets off a round of fire into the air and everyone becomes hysterical.

No one seems to know what is going on or what this man is wanting. It turns into a state of chaos, with people running about like mice in a cage. Then the armed man just states that nobody would be going anywhere until he got what he wanted.

I don't get to hear what his demands are because the doctors are now trying to work out how they are going to get to the main part of the hospital where the dialysis machine was kept. The three of them argue about who is going to make a run for it without the shooter seeing them. Clare states it is too dangerous to go now and they will just have to wait it out until the situation has resolved. Dr A agrees but could see how I was deteriorating and may not be able to wait that long. Dr L is shouting that I need to be on dialysis now and can't wait any longer.

Some of the men in the crowd are looking in at us through the window and can see the dire state going on in my room. Then a few men start making a ruckus to distract the shooter and then one gave the doctors a nod of his head to say to go now. Just like that, Dr L opens the door and darts out of the building and around the back, then sprints towards the main part of the hospital. The shooter is too distracted with the decoy going on to notice Dr L escape. I just had to wait and hold on a little longer until I could get on dialysis to keep my body alive.

It is a very hot day. The temperature outside has climbed to 40 degrees Celsius. My room is in a separate building outside of the main hospital and the air conditioning doesn't seem to be working well at all. The room is quite small and has chairs along two sides of it with a small palm in a pot in one corner. Geoff is here visiting, along with my other brother, Eddie. The two are sweltering now and as the nurse walks in, Geoff asks her if she could turn up the air conditioning. She replies that it is regulated by the main hospital and she has no control over it. I can see the sweat trickling down the side of his and Eddie's faces. I'm not too affected by the heat, I have got used to having a warm room with the various treatments I had been having.

Geoff keeps walking over to the temperature control saying it was now reading 41 degrees and this was ridiculous. Then, through the big glass window that overlooked the car park entrance, Geoff sees Les and my son Mark driving through the boom gates in my blue Tucson Hyundai SUV.

Five minutes later, Les and Mark arrive and greet me with a kiss on the cheek. After some idle chat between them, Les and Mark soon begin to wilt in the heat too. Mark has my yellow iPhone and asks me if I want to listen to my 70s and 80s play list? I tell him that would be nice and he sets it playing quietly in the background. I always like to have music on at home all day, music is a huge part of my life, it uplifts me. The temperature seems to be climbing and I can see Mark really struggling with the heat. I keep repeating please go home to all of them, it is just too hot to visit on a day like this.

Les can see how Mark is being affected by the intense heat, so agrees to take him home. I tell Mark to take the phone with him and he could bring it back next time. Geoff decides to go as well and I am relieved. I feel bad they have come to visit me on such a blisteringly hot day. Eddie says he will stay a little longer until the nurse comes back so that I'm not alone in these harsh conditions.

After the three of them had left, the nurse walks in to do my obs. Eddie is sitting there watching when he gets a call from Les saying Mark had dropped the phone at the boom gates as they were driving and could he go and pick it up before somebody else finds it? Eddie passes on the message to me and says he will be back after he has picked up the phone. I watch him walk out and through the window, I can see him out at the boom gates retrieving the phone.

The nurse is finishing off my obs when the door bursts open with a sudden force. We both turn to look in surprise at the noise and in comes the shooter with his weapon still on him. We are both startled by his sudden entrance and too dumbfounded to do or say anything. He makes his way to the front of my bed and stands there in a dictatorial manner, tall and strong with his eyes staring unwaveringly. He tells me no one will be leaving or entering my room until I had confessed and given him all the details about the conspiracy order. The nurse tells him she needs to get my medication or I will die. He states he doesn't care and will do whatever he has to do to get the information out of me.

Eddie, standing outside in the blisteringly hot sun can see what is happening inside. He holds up the phone and starts to play my list from Spotify, his way of letting me know he is going to get help and not to do anything. I keep looking at Eddie, who is sweating intensely out in the oppressive midday heat. I can hear the music playing. As the shooter turns around to find out where the music is coming from, the nurse gives me a sign she is going to do something about it. I whisper that Eddie is signalling that he has it under control and to leave it up to him. The shooter, still intent on what Eddie is doing as he is waving the phone around in the air, is trying to figure out what his intention is.

Both the nurse and I keep our eyes on the shooter while silently communicating with each other, planning on doing different strategies. I beg her not to do anything and let Eddie take care of it all. She doesn't believe he can do anything without help and she must go and try and do something before it is too late. Feeling very panicked now, as I knew Eddie had a plan and she would most likely ruin it, I watch as she makes a start to the door but the shooter turns around sees her move away. The hospital has another part of it I haven't come across before. My room is at the end of an alley that is very cosmopolitan-like mixed with a gypsy camp feel. The lane has a lot of food markets under canvas tops, all with different types of food to try. There are lampposts like those you would see in the 1600s–the ones that had a metal cage to hold a small fire that burned slowly to light the area. Music is being played by small groups of musicians with a singer. The music is lively and people are dancing free and easy with their hands in the air and wide smiles on their happy faces. Trees line the dirt alley with lots of dark shadowy spots where the fire lanterns can't illuminate the way. It is a balmy night with a breeze gently whisking past just enough to cool your skin and keep you feeling comfortable.

Clare is looking after me again in my small cosy cottage room. It has a wooden door with a window either side. The windows each have four panes and are big enough for you to be able to get glimpses of the top half of the passers-by in the alleyway. I can hear the music playing along with the mumbled sounds of people's conversations and the merriment going on.

Thud, thud, thud is heard on top of the thatched roof. Both Clare and I look up at the ceiling to try and work out what the sound is. As it continues, it becomes very agitating like a dripping tap. We can both see people starting to gather outside my room and are looking up to the roof top. Eddie is out there observing what is going on when Clare decides to walk outside and check it out for herself.

There, crouched on the thatched roof is this little man. He is dwarf-sized and wearing brown pants with a red and white checked shirt. He has short brown hair with a goatee and bright brown eyes that set off his face. He is holding a metal mace which he relentlessly pounds on the roof. He isn't speaking or indicating what he wants, just in a state totally unaware of the people gathered around.

Clare tells the crowd to leave so she can work out how to resolve the problem. As the crowd slowly move on, Eddie asks Clare if she wants him to do something to get rid of the small man. She tells him to just wait a little longer to see if he leaves on his own accord. After a short time, both Clare and I are on the verge of mental distraction, the constant thudding getting on our nerves. Clare goes outside to Eddie, telling him to do whatever he needed to do to get the man off the roof. Eddie says he will go and get his twin brother, who was now up on a ward in the hospital to help him.

Before long, Eddie returns with our brother, Will. Will was always *an overwhelming presence to those who did not know him. Tall and robust in stature with a big burly voice and a moustache. But for those who knew him, he was just a giant teddy bear who was very protective of his family. So there they are, standing side by side like brothers-in-arms ready to fight a battle to protect their little sister as they had always done throughout their life.*

Clare tells them if they need anything, she can acquire black market items, anything at all, no matter what it takes to resolve the issue. On hearing this through the walls, I suddenly have a different perception of Clare and can't help but wonder if she wasn't part of this conspiracy thing after all. I had to keep my doubts to myself, now fearing my own safety with Clare looking after me.

The thudding is ceaseless and it was obvious the boys are unable to entice the man off the roof. There is a knock on the door, so Clare walks over to open it. With the door ajar, I overhear the conversation between my brothers and Clare. They ask her if they can go to the next level of intervention. Clare goes over to her desk and on a piece of paper, writes the name and number of a contact who would be able to supply them with whatever they needed. As she hands over the note, my brothers inquire, 'Anything?' She nods, answering, 'Yes.' My brothers look at each other with excitement and quickly start on their way. Clare shuts the door and walks back in without any change to her persona. All I can think is how cool and calculating she is.

Within a few hours, my brothers return. I can vaguely hear them trying to make a deal with the small man. Clare and I look at each other with surprise and relief, the thudding had finally stopped. Clare goes outside to see what the boys had done but no one is out there. We just have to wait for them to return to find out what the resolution involved.

It isn't too long before they return and with the door ajar again, I overhear the boys saying they obtained some sawn-off shot guns, some heavy chains and a few other weapons. I can't believe what I am hearing. Surely, they wouldn't have killed the man. That was not like my brothers. NO. It couldn't be true. Then I hear them say to Clare that if there were any other jobs to be done, they would be happy to oblige. She tells them there could be another job soon and to stay in touch. I am confounded and totally bewildered by the events that have just occurred.

Will is standing outside my door calling out to Clare. Clare walks outside to see what Will wants and through the open door I see my brother standing there, big and strong but in a restless state. I had seen him like this before when he was taking hard drugs. He is swaying and fidgeting like a lion trapped in a cage. Clare asks him what he did with the dwarf man. Will tells her he and Eddie had taken him out to the wood and shot him, then chopped him up into little pieces and disposed of him in a big drum of acid to dissolve his body.

I am shocked to hear this. Surely, he wouldn't do such an atrocious crime. As I am processing this, I observe Clare and she doesn't seem to be phased by this at all. I quickly realise she is definitely part of the conspiracy. Any normal person wouldn't react like that. I now I have doubts about Will.

I begin to wonder where Eddie is, he and Will are always together, like most twins tended to be. This can't really be happening. Then I hear Clare asks Will the same thing. He proudly looks down to the ground where there is now a canvas covering something. Will says Eddie was getting too out of hand and wanted to do even worse things than he would consider and has become too dangerous. Will lifts the canvas to reveal pieces of Eddie's limbs and torso topped with his severed head, stating that he had to take care of him. Will laughs at how funny Eddie looks. Clare just stares at Will, no expression at all on her face and Will's bellowing laugh echoes through my disbelieving mind. How could he do that to his twin brother? Eddie was a good, kind-hearted and loving brother. This cannot be happening.

Next thing, I am in the same vicinity of the alley but around a bend, which widens into another open-air area with similar lighting. Fires are spotted throughout, with groups of people sitting around talking, eating, drinking and enjoying themselves. I have been wheeled down on my bed by the South African nurse as we had been told I would be next on the list for surgery. The operating theatres are down in this area, so we just have to wait until they are ready. There I am, lying in a critical state. I know I'm not at all well and feel myself going in and out of consciousness. Hon is with me. She is soothingly stroking the top of my head while she plays my 'feeling swanky' playlist on Spotify.

I feel very exposed and vulnerable as I lay there with people casually walking by doing their own thing, totally oblivious of me. I am comforted by Hon gently caressing my head, though, and hearing my favourite songs in the background.

The South African nurse keeps moving away from the bed and I start to wonder what she is doing. Then Hon tells me there is a small person, like a hobbit, who keeps coming over to the bed and being a real distraction and annoyance. The nurse is trying to get rid of him as he bounces around like a boxer going into the ring to fight. Dancing around, saying inaudible words and hovering around my bed. The nurse, who usually talked in a kind voice, now has a vexed tone. She moves over towards him and repeatedly kicks him hard and I could feel myself becoming unnerved. After repeatedly booting the hobbit, he scurries off like a whimpering dog with its tail between its legs.

The nurse returns, becoming impatient with the hold up with the surgery. I should have been done an hour ago. I too am becoming anxious about the delay. You mentally prepare for what's about to happen but the longer the delay, the more worry sets in. The nurse leaves to find out what is going on. Hon is still with me, so I feel a little reassured.

The nurse re-joins us and is furious. She announces that I must be taken back to the ward as the surgeons had been held up and wouldn't have time to do me. She says she had told them I had been waiting for hours and that I was in a critical state but the doctors said I would just have to wait until tomorrow. I am gutted. Am I really that unimportant? Shoved to the back of the list when I had been waiting so long already. Being totally dismayed in my helpless state, the nurse wheels me back to my room.

Now, as I came in and out of consciousness I become aware of my surroundings. I can sense I am in that outdoor area again, the smells and sounds familiar only, this time I have a metal grate covering my body about 4 cm above. Then I see the surgeon standing above my head looking down over me in his white gown and mask. He announces I would have the surgery now and asks if I am still willing to go ahead with it. I nod my head, yes.

GGGGRRRRRRR is the loud sound the angle grinder makes as the surgeon starts it up. Looking directly above me through the metal grate I can see the power tool slowly come closer towards me. I am wide awake; no anaesthetic has been given to me. What the hell are they thinking? Panic rises in me like a tidal wave. I try yelling out but my voice can't be heard above the sound of the angle grinder.

Sparks begin to fly as the grinding teeth of the power bite into the metal grate. The sparks are bright red and orange and the smell of metal teeth gnashing on the metal grate is like nothing else. The assault on my olfactory senses is intense, to say the least, but that tidal wave of panic is now one of sheer terror. What will happen once the protective grate covering me can no longer hold the mighty assault by this metal demon?

I am standing in a small clearing in the forest area near the hospital down South. It is a beautiful sunny day and everything is *so peaceful as I stand there enjoying the wooded surrounds. Geoff shows up with his shotgun and greets me in a welcoming and friendly manner. I am pleased to see him and as he comes closer, reach out to him and he gives me a huge hug. I ask him what he is doing and he replies that he's going into the woods to do some hunting. It is his way of getting away from things, he finds being in the densely wooded area and the excitement of looking for game calming. I smile at him and wish him good luck with his hunt, then wave him goodbye as he heads into the forest.*

Not long after Geoff leaves, Will and Eddie rock up. They don't have the calm nature that Geoff had expressed, they are both quite highly strung, fidgeting and bouncing around on their feet. They ask if I'm going to join the conspiracy movement. I look at them in astonishment. 'Why do you ask such a question?'

'Well, if you're not going to, we are going into the forest after Geoff and kill him,' Will responds.

'Why are you into this conspiracy thing? This is not like you boys. You're all brothers, blood kin. You can't kill him,' I answer back.

'Sis, it's all up to you. If you come over to our side then everything will be OK. We'll even let Les, Scott and Mark go. They are still alive but time is running out.'

'You know where Les and the boys are being kept?' I respond in a panic.

Of course, we put them there. They're all tied up in your pool with their heads above water, the dinghy over top of them. I imagine they will be getting pretty cold by now and soon they will run out of energy and sink and drown.' Will's voice is so cold.

I can't believe what I'm hearing from my own brothers. How they could kill my own family so coldly and callously. What is the point of having the heart transplant if I have no one to share my life with? This can't be true. My mind is in turmoil.

'We will then go up to Mum and kill her too,' Will states.

'Why Mum? She is your own mother. Why do you have to kill her? She hasn't done anything wrong.'

'She is old and has no more purpose in life, so after your family is dead, then we will go up and kill her too. We found out where Stephen had been. We know where the rehab centre is and are going to kill him too."

'You can't go and kill Stephen. He is finally trying to get himself straight and sorted out. He is getting on the right path and has a chance of having a good life.' I say despairingly.

'Well come over to our side and none of this will have to happen, then we can convert all of your family as well and they will be under our control too,' Will replies.

I can't make sense of all the information swirling in my head. If I go over to the conspiracy then none of us will have any control of our own lives and if I don't, then everyone I love will be dead. And I know it isn't just us but the whole world who would be at risk of being overtaken by this world dominion. What did that eventually mean? I am obviously important to them but why? Maybe I am the one who, for some reason, can bring them down. I have to fight them.

As I am blankly staring ahead with these thoughts processing in my mind, Will says, 'Well, looks like we're going on a hunt after Geoff and then up to your house to take care of things up there.' My blank gaze turns to one of horror as I watch them run into the woods calling for Geoff.

'No, no. Not Geoff.' I scream out for Geoff to keep running, hearing the boys howling like wild banshees rounding up wild pigs. BANG. A gunshot resounds. But whose?

I wake up in my room after the surgery and I hear the voices of my family. I am still in a very drowsy state and just can't bring myself to open my eyes but can clearly hear everything that is being said. I hear Scott telling Les and Mark how he had come off his motorbike and broken his thumb. He was retelling how the accident happened but other than his thumb, he wasn't hurt in any other way. Hearing this conversation, I am confused about the details. As far as I knew Scott only had a car licence and is still on his 'P' plates. He never had a bike licence or a bike for that matter. Surely, he hasn't gone and obtained his licence without me knowing? Has he sold his car to get his motor bike? He'd only just finished doing his car up. Surely not?

I am recovering after the surgery but the room I am in has wooden floors and is in an upstairs level. The window looks outside over a lake and seems to be isolated from anything else. I have an intubation tube down my throat which seems to have a middle lever in the centre part of my mouth. The mouthpiece has a centre bar that almost reaches the bottom section leaving just enough leeway to be able to move the lever to either side of it. I can't talk or even move my head, for that matter. The South African nurse is again looking after me but her manner is slightly hostile. I feel apprehensive.

As she strides towards me in a belligerent manner, my guard goes up. She starts asking me questions about the little hobbit man that was hanging around my bed when I was waiting for the surgery.

'You knew him, didn't you? He is part of your group isn't he? He was trying to get you to tell him something, perhaps a plan against the conspiracy?' she says.

'No, I don't know him at all,' I whisper, my voice hoarse and struggling to make any sound at all.

'Then why was he hovering nearby and wouldn't go away?' she replies. I just nod my head side-to-side slightly as it is too hard to try and talk. 'I know you were trying to pass on plans to him. Why else would a person like him be wanting to come near you?' I again nod my head sideways in a pleading manner. My eyes are focused on her and welling up with tears. 'Can't talk, hey? How about we move this lever to the other side, maybe then you might be able to say something?' she says vindictively. Leaning over me, she begins to forcibly push down on the metal lever with all her weight to try and manoeuvre it below the small gap at the bottom of the centre bar. It is really uncomfortable as she forces the lever across to the other side. It feels as if a dentist is levering a molar from my mouth. I grimace as she proceeds but am not going to give her the pleasure of knowing how much it hurts.

'Now let's see if you can talk. Tell me what you were planning to tell him? Or else I have your Pet dog Jasper and I will take great pleasure in pulling his teeth out one by one.' Her voice menacing. Once again, I try to shout out but only a hoarse whisper comes out. I am fearful of what she might do to my poor little Jasper if she really did get hold of him. 'I can see that you really can't speak because of the intubation tube. Well, perhaps I should go and put it back to the other side since it doesn't seem to make any difference,' she says in a masochistic tone. My adrenalin levels rise as I watch her lower herself down toward me with a sinister grin on her face.

My room now has two doctors, along with Clare and the South African nurse. I am still in the isolated upstairs room and can see the view out of the large window overlooking the lake, which is as calm as a mill pond. Then I hear my brother's voice, Will.

As Will keeps bellowing out, the nurses and doctors move over to the window to see what all the noise is about. I can see the backs of them as they peer out the window but can only just make out Will's head. I hear him yelling he's coming to save me. 'You can't stop me. I know what you're trying to do to my sister and I'm going to come and get her. You can't stop me.'

'Seems like your brother is going to be a problem,' Clare states, turning around and looking at me. As the doctors keep watching,

Will makes his way towards the stairs. 'Call security,' Dr A says to the South African nurse. I hear her talking to security to come and resolve the situation.

Thud, thud, thud go the sound of Will's heavy footsteps as he climbs the stairs. Then grappling and thumping with the muffled sounds of men tackling each other. Security manages to pull Will down the stairs and send him on his way. The medical staff move away from the window as the disturbance settles, chatting amongst themselves in low enough voices so that I can't hear. Then the bellowing starts up again. The doctors and nurses once again go to the window and I hear Clare say, 'He's got a gun. Shall I call for the next level of intervention?' Dr A nods his head. As Clare strides past me she mutters, 'Your brother is quite a problem,' in a sneering tone. My brothers are very protective of me and have always been but I didn't think Will would go this far.

After several moments, I hear police sirens wailing outside on the road. Clare announced that two policemen with automatic rifles and hand-held guns are walking towards Will. I hear the police tell him to put down the gun.

'No, not until I've got my little sister out,' Will yells.

BANG. Another gunshot but who shot it? I'm feeling quite worried for Will, I know he will not give up easily. Will then lets out a retaliating shot followed by the deafening BBBBrrrrrr of the police automatic weapons. Then SPLASH– the sound of Will falling backwards into the water. Then silence.

'OK, well looks like that's been taken care of,' Clare says in a matter-of-fact way. The doctors let out a sigh of relief in unison and turn away from the window when a mumbled bellowing begins again.

What is happening? How can they all be so cold and callous about this? Will is my brother and they're treating him like an annoying fly that needs to be swatted.

'Is that all you've got?' Will bellows as he rises out of the water. 'A few bullet holes aren't going to do anything to me. Remember, I've taken a lot of drugs in my time and become pretty bullet-proof. What else you got, huh?'

The doctors and nurses look at each other, astonished at what they are seeing.

'How can he be standing with bullet holes all through him?' Clare asks in disbelief.

'He's not normal, no human could take what he's just had done to him,' Dr A states.

'Come on. I'm coming to get my little sis.' Will confidently shouts.

The staff watch through the window as Will defiantly strides out of the water. 'Unbelievable,' Clare says, followed by the deafening sound of the automatic rounds once again being fired. SPLASH! Like the sound of a cut-down tree falling into the water. Poor Will. My truly loyal brother has been felled once again. Surely, he can't take any more of this unjust battle. He needs to just stay down.

'Ha ha ha!' Will's laugh echoes.

'For God's sake, bring in the military,' Clare barks as she marches over to the phone.

Her face is red, pupils dilated, enraged. 'They're on their way with the chopper,' she says as she hangs up the phone. As she paces past me, she glares. Clare is seething now and I have no idea of what she is capable of doing.

'Here I come,' Will mocks. His body now looking like Swiss cheese, he slowly and deliberately walks out of the water again.

'Shit,' Dr A announces in bewilderment.

Then comes the heavy sound of the chopper blades moving

closer. What are they going to do now? The thundering noise is terrifying as the helicopter hovers just above Will's head.

'Come on. Try me,' he shouts at the chopper. Then the giant bird of prey slowly lowers itself on to the target, I can hear the splashing of water as the giant blades whip at it like a beater whipping up egg whites. What the hell do they think they're going to do to him? He's a human being after all, not some prehistoric T-rex.

Jesus, I think to myself, watching them all ogling at the giant metal bird as it lowered itself in front of us.

Will, standing with his arms reaching up to the predator and waiting for it to come into contact to tackle it, yells at it in a battle charge command like the Hulk in his green, angered state. Then, his mighty sound begins to gurgle as he is pushed below the water's surface. Hovering in place for what seemed like eternity with nothing but its thunderous whirling blades to be heard, the mighty bird then slowly begins to retreat upwards.

'Oh my God!' Dr A exclaims.

'I don't believe it. That's impossible,' Clare says, astonished as they watch Will once again rise out of the water like a phoenix rising from the ashes.

'Come again, you bastard,' Will bellows to the chopper.

Down sinks the chopper, hovering over its target until the sound of Will's voice falls silent. This time, the metal bird stays in place longer, holding Will beneath the watery depths devoid of life-giving oxygen.

Eventually, the helicopter retreats to the heavens. No sounds. Nothing. All of us waiting with bated breath for it to return but only deathly silence echoes in our ears.

Still in the same room over the lake, I don't know what to expect after the barbaric assault on Will. The South African nurse is still taking care of me and Clare seems to be regularly waltzing in and out of my room. Two doctors, along with an Indian nurse with long black hair, are also in here. The mood is quite different to anything I have experienced before. Everyone is in an exhilarated sexualised state, carrying on in an outlandish manner and being flamboyant with each other. It is totally bizarre.

Clare enters the room wearing a skimpy French maid's outfit, black fish net stockings with stilettos and talking in a high pitch as she bounds over to a locked cupboard. Unlocking it and retrieving a black tube, she announces, 'I need a black hit.'

'But you've just had a purple one less than an hour ago. I think you've had enough for a while,' says one of the doctors.

'I don't care, I'm so aroused but I need to get higher,' Clare responds, jittery.

I watch her bend over and stick this black suppository tube in her rectum. Standing upright, she is overcome with a rush of ecstasy and arousal, totally out of control and buzzing around the doctors and nurses.

Glancing over towards me lying on a mattress on the floor, she advances. 'You are no better than your brother. You are just like him. I bet you are just putting on all this pretence,' she says, snarling.

Curled up in a foetal position, I don't even try to respond. It would be no use anyway.

'I think we need to give her a black dose and see if she responds to it like her brothers Eddie and Will did. They absolutely loved taking these drugs. They really knew how to party and have a good time on them. Give her one and let's see if she can control herself, or wants to party like her brothers,' Clare tells the Indian nurse. Clare glares at me, turns around then skips across the floor and exits the room.

The Indian nurse does as she was told. Having a black

suppository now in her hand, she inserts it in my rectum. However, she isn't like Clare or the South African nurse, who are obviously part of this conspiracy. She seems genuinely concerned and upset for me. Watching me as tears stream down my face, her eyes hold my distressed gaze in sympathy.

After half an hour and with me not having any response to the inserted drug, she quietly says, 'So you're not part of this conspiracy?'

'No, I'm here just to have a heart transplant. I don't do drugs or any of that sort of stuff that my brothers do,' My tone one of hopelessness.

'So, you're not getting any sexual arousal at all?' she asks.

'No, none at all but none of them will believe me,' I answer.

'I believe you. I'll try and talk them into letting you go with all this conspiracy ordeal,' she says eagerly. I can tell she sincerely did believe me and I only hope now that she may be able to make them finally see sense.

Still in my isolated room overlooking the lake, some time has passed since the devastating event with my brother, Will but I can't say how long as time seems to be irrelevant in this world I am now existing in. I'm still recovering from the heart transplant and know I'm not doing very well but at least I am still alive, which means there is hope of getting out of here.

'We've got your mother coming to visit you. Perhaps she may be able to talk some sense into you and get you to realise who you really are in the conspiracy order,' announces Clare as she saunters towards me in a contemptuous manner. She wistfully plays with and flicks my bedding pretending to neaten it up. 'Let's see what sense she can talk into you,' she continues before turning and walking out the door.

I am left lying here, bewildered once again. When will this

nonsense stop? Mum will be able to get me out of here or at least get some help. Someone that is not part of this stupid conspiracy thing, I think to myself.

Mum is driving down the road toward the hospital room. She gets out of the car and heads towards my room but is intercepted by a tall man wearing a brown tailored suit and a Fedora. Startled by his sudden appearance, she stops and looks up at him. 'Oh, I didn't see you there before. You've taken me by surprise, sorry,' says Mum, startled.

'Sorry, I never meant to startle you. It's just that you seem to be heading over toward the room ahead. The staff there asked me to stop you coming in as things have taken a turn for the worse with your daughter and they need to work on her. They will give you a call later and let you know how things are going when they've finished,' answers the man. Seeming distressed by the news, Mum turns around and goes back to her car, worrying about what had gone wrong with me.

As I hear the car drive off, I am thinking, NO. Come back, Mum. What are you doing? She was my only hope and now she's gone. My mind is spinning around in a million circles trying to figure this whole calamity out but nothing is making any sense.

Just then, the door bursts open and the surgeon waltzes towards me and states in a commanding voice, 'We couldn't let your mother in as we know she hasn't any clue about the conspiracy and we can't risk her finding out about us. So we've made a decision. We've got someone coming in that you may know and if you can tell us who he is, then we'll let you off on this conspiracy interrogation.' Once again, I am dumbfounded but have no choice but to go along with it.

Before long, a tall man wearing a brown sheriff's uniform with a silver star badge pinned to his shirt above the left pocket enters the room. A cream Texan hat crowns his head and teardrop sunglasses cover his eyes, highlighting his rosy chubby cheeks. I watch as he approaches, wondering who he is and why I should know him.

'How ya doin' there, Mam?' he asks in a Texan drawl.

Unsure of what to say, I give him my normal response, 'I'm good thanks.'

'I've been asked to come in and ask you a few questions about your brothers being in the woods the other day?' he says.

Looking a little stunned, trying to figure out how he knew about them being out there that day, I sit there just staring at him.

'I heard via the grapevine that there was an incident.'

'I don't know anything about that. What makes you think I would know?' The colour drains from my face as I try and conceal my lies.

'Well, somebody said they saw you out there that day. They described you and your three brothers quite clearly.'

Watching his unwavering gaze, I am really feeling very uncomfortable now. Not wanting to say anything as it would incriminate me, I just sit there and re-confirm, 'I really don't know what you're talking about.'

The sheriff moves away from my bed and heads over to the doctors to talk to them. As I lay there not looking over toward them to avoid looking concerned, I strain my ears to try and hear what they are talking about.

Then the sheriff returns. 'Well that will be all for now. I'll be back to ask more questions another time.' As he speaks,, something about him seems vaguely familiar but I can't put my finger on it. Why does he seem familiar?

The next day, the South African nurse returns to look after me. As she comes into my room, I know this isn't going to be good.

'So, you still refuse to acknowledge you are part of our

conspiracy. Well yesterday was proof to us that you are. You didn't even recognise your own eldest brother,' she says, sneering.

Quizzically looking at her, my brain is back tracking to the sheriff but I can't believe he is David. He had a Yankee accent and why would he pose as a sheriff, for God's sake?

The nurse, watching the blank stare on my face confirms, 'Yes, that was your brother. He's part of us as well. That means you are in the conspiracy because when anyone enters we wipe the memory of their family from their mind. You couldn't recognise him and that's proof enough for us.'

'Well then, how come he knew who I was if our memories are wiped? That doesn't make sense.' I say defensively.

'Oh, once you've been on a probation period we can re-instate them back into your memories. Your brother has been with us for a long time,' she answers.

I know my brother too well; he would never be corrupted to the other side. He just wouldn't. This conspiracy order must have some extremely potent drugs to infiltrate even the most honest people without them knowing. I really can't let them weave themselves into society any further.

Who am I kidding? I'm only one insignificant person. There is really nothing I can do. I am now realising the detriment of this whole crisis.

'Well, we've got a little way of making you remember,' she says in a jovial tone accompanied by a huge grin. She forces a little black pill down my throat.

Wondering what the hell she has just given me, my eyes wide with fear, she grabs me and walks me over to a door that opens out above the lake. I never noticed it before. As she opens the door, a gang plank appears leading to deeper water.

Roughly tying my hands behind my back, she says, smirking, 'I think you're going to enjoy this.'

We reach the end of the long bridge. The platform at the end is quite a dizzying height as I peer down over the edge. Surely she must just be bluffing. She's not going to push me off. Someone will find out. She can't be that insane.

Cold grips my body as bubbles flow up past my face. The murky blue water stabbing my bare skin with its icy nettles. The light from the sun begins to dim as the watery depths seem to go on forever. I don't know how long I was down there but my breath never seemed to run out. I wait for the gasping for life to begin but it is like everything is running in slow motion. Cold, empty darkness surrounds me. What is happening? Have I died and don't know it? Why hasn't someone come and retrieved my body? Is this purgatory that I'm in? Then the fight for life grips me like nothing I had ever experienced before. I begin thrashing about trying to wriggle free from the bonds that hold me down. My urge for air is an explosion of panic like an atomic bomb going off inside me. I am going to die. Hell, no one will ever know what they've done to me. Slowly my movements slow and a calmness overtakes my writhing body. All becomes peaceful as the watery vision surrounding turns black.

Bright lights are blinding me and my chest is racked with pain as I take a huge gasp of air and then vomit the water filling my stomach.

'There, I told you, you would like it. Fun isn't it?' the South African nurse says, smiling. What sick minded person would do that to anyone? I think to myself, still recovering from the traumatic ordeal I had just been through.

'There we go, you can rest now, everything is alright.' She fusses about tucking me in bed as if she really cares for me.

I am numb.

Clare merrily waltzes in and says to the South African nurse, 'Give me a pill, surprise me with the colour, too. Don't show me it.'

The nurse hands her a pill and says, 'Shut your eyes so you don't peek at the colour.'

Clare obediently closes her eyes and swallows. Excitedly, she opens the hidden door I had been through and eagerly says, 'Tie me up. Come on, I can't wait. I love doing this.'

The nurse, excited too, ties Clare's hands behind her back. They are acting like two schoolgirls mucking about together, giggling and playing. Then Clare hurries along the bridge to the end platform and jumps off.

What the hell is she doing? No one in their right mind would willingly do that. This was crazy.

The South African nurse prances around my room trying to hold back her glee. 'Ooh. Isn't this just wonderful?' she says, oozing with excitement.

I stare blankly at her, not knowing what to answer. The door bursts open and a dripping wet Clare staggers through.

Looking dishevelled and gasping for her breath, she says, 'Jeez, I love the adrenalin rush of doing that.' Regaining her composure, she stands up straight, still dripping wet and says, 'How did you like your first time Colleen?'

I don't answer.

Another nurse comes in and the South African nurse says to her, 'Here, take this pill.'

The other nurse looks at her quizzically but does as she's told.

Watching what was transpiring before me, I am still trying to figure out what their whole plan is. The new nurse doesn't seem too phased about was occurring, as if she'd been through it before but was seems reluctant. But with her hands tied behind her back, she *follows the same procedure and walks along the bridge.*

Sometime later, the South African nurse says to Clare, 'I had better go and get her.'

Clare nods her head.

On returning, Clare says to the South African nurse, 'Where is she?'

'Oh, she was a pain in the arse. She never did like doing this with us. I gave her a purple pill instead. She never did appreciate what we do.'

'Where did you put her body?' Clare asks.

'There is a medical dumpster out the back. No one ever looks in there because of the hazard waste disposed in it,' she replies.

'Good thinking,' Clare agrees.

Morning comes around before I know it. I am exhausted by all the hideous events that have occurred. Too tired to even try and think about what is going to play out next.

In a cheerful voice, the South African nurse says, 'Good morning, Colleen. How are we feeling today? Ready for another exciting day of fun?'

Eyeing her off warily, I stay silent.

'Now, now, we don't have to be like that. It doesn't take much to be pleasant now, does it?' she says sarcastically.

Clare enters my room with a bounce in her step. 'All righty then, are we ready to go?'

'I think we are. Ready as she'll ever be,' the South African nurse replies while looking at me. 'Here we go. Pop this in your mouth now.' She passes me a pill.

'No, I'm not taking it. You're both insane,' I say. But between the two of them they manage to hold me down and force it down my throat.

'It didn't have to be that hard, now, did it? You're making it difficult and unpleasant. You should be a good girl and do as you're told,' the South African nurse says angrily.

I am once again consumed with fear, not knowing what pill they gave me. Either way, I'll go through the terror as I did yesterday or end up dead like the other nurse and be thrown in the dumpster. Fighting all the way down the bridge, I try to push back against the nurse to stop moving forward.

'No use fighting. You'll get used to it after a while. We do this regularly and love it. You will too, just wait and see,' the South African nurse tells me, shoving me forward.

What do you mean, I'll get used to it? How many times do they think they're going to do this to me? I can't keep going through this. For God's sake, will somebody come and save me? I think to myself as she pushes me off the platform.

Lying in bed recovering from the transplant, Mark asks me what Spotify playlist did I want to listen to? Unable to answer because I'm still semi-conscious, he tells me he will put on my 70s and 80s playlist. I can hear the old familiar songs, which is comforting. Even though I am lying in bed, I am mentally transported into an interrogation room at the conspiracy headquarters.

'You know why we know you are part of us? It's because you play Spotify all the time and that is the real-world control centre. Everyone who listens to Spotify is under our control,' a woman dressed in a pencil skirt, blouse and black high heeled shoes says. She has blonde hair tied back into a ponytail and red lipstick. Her uniform is a greyish green colour and she reminds me of the Nazi regime you saw in old movies. 'You love Spotify and you're always playing music from it and creating playlists. The control centre can *track everything you do and where you go from you using this app,' she continues.*

'No, I just use Spotify like millions of other people around the world because it's the best music app you can get,' I reply. 'You can't tell me millions of people are already under your control without knowing about it.'

'That's where you're wrong. They are under our control and soon we'll have world domination, you just wait and see,' she replies. 'Every time you play Spotify, we know exactly what you're doing and where you are and even better, we can mind control you by subliminally putting codes and thoughts into songs,' I woman continues, outwardly impressed with the depth of control they seemed to have over people.

Now dumbfounded by the level of control the conspiracy seems to have, I am starting to feel a real threat. Just how deep are they in and what level of control do they really have? What is their goal once complete control has been achieved? These thoughts rattle through my brain like an out-of-control freight train racing down the track. This is beyond me. My mind is at a standstill, not able to think at all, completely blank. All I know is I can't play Spotify anymore. I have to stop Mark from playing it for me and tell others not to use it either. I'm getting agitated, Mark is playing the music. I must try and stop him and get the phone away from me.

It is the mid-1800s, around the time of the Boer War in South Africa. We are in a camp with the British with large white tents erected into a settlement. Everyone is dressed in the clothing of that time. Men are in trousers, buttoned up white shirts and tailored coats while the women wear ankle-length layered petticoat dresses with long sleeves. Our campsite is on the Savannah out in the open with just long dried grasses thinly scattered, wisping in the wind. I am heavily pregnant but now suffering complications which needed medical

intervention. I am lying on a bed in the medical tent with a nurse and a doctor with a thick, short black beard and who is very thin in stature.

'Well now, we have to intubate you to get the fluid out of your lungs. This procedure may not be particularly comfortable but it has to be done or you may die from pneumonia and your baby will also die in utero,' the doctor announces to me as he prepares the tubing and instruments.

The nurse is fussing around me saying, 'Everything will be alright; the doctor knows what he's doing.'

I don't feel reassured by the amount of nervous energy she seems to have, showing very little confidence.

The nurse is told to hold me down as the doctor inserts the tube down my throat. I'm not sure of what to expect as this is not a common procedure for this time and I'm tensing myself up ready to fight.

As the doctor tells me to open my mouth and just take deep breaths, the most invasive and gut-wrenching feeling overtakes me. My breath comes in gasping fits as the invading predator forces its way down my airway. Things are not meant to go down this tube, it's like going against the laws of nature. My body is trying to repel this intrusive being but it is a battle it wasn't going to win. Then a calmness takes over, the convulsions of my body easing.

'There we go. Only uncomfortable for a moment then, wasn't it?' the doctor says in a patronising tone.

I'm lying there with this tube down my throat and can't talk.

The nurse then takes another tube and, hovering over me, says, 'Now this won't be anywhere as bad as the main intubation tube being inserted. This one just slides down inside the main pipe and then we can suck out any fluid that is in your lungs.'

Even though I am still a bit hesitant as she leans over and begins the insertion, I realise she was right; I didn't feel it. After hearing some sucking and slurping noises as the fluid was being excreted from my lungs, I can still feel this invasive probing deep within my lungs. It's not a feeling I ever want to get used to.

After the draining of my lungs, the doctor says to the nurse, 'We can pull out the intubation tube now nurse. Can you just come over in case I need you to hold Colleen still?'

She comes over and when he's about to pull the tube out, he says to me, 'Now just keep blowing out until I say stop.'

Then this weird feeling inside me starts rising as the invasive intruder is evacuated from my body. But then the rising feeling in my stomach couldn't be contained and I vomit all over myself.

The nurse politely cleans me up and says, 'Never mind, that's quite normal. Don't worry about it.' She is very comforting to me.

I sleep comfortably that night and feel reasonably well, except for a little coughing. When the doctor comes in to check me the next morning, he listens to my chest with his stethoscope.

Looking a little worried, he says to me, 'Sorry, but we are going to have to intubate again and drain out more fluid which has built up over night.'

I really don't want to go through that procedure again. The horrible, invasive feeling of something going down the wrong way.

Before I can get my thoughts together and prepare myself for the assault that is going to happen to my body, the doctor and nurse are hovering over me. The nurse's hands grip my head like a vice as the doctor begins to force the tube down my throat. I am writhing and squirming, trying to avoid the awful invasion to my lungs. I am fighting it all the way. Not being able to breathe, the gag reflex kicks in, as do the spasms in my stomach. I feel like my insides are convulsing but the vice grip on my head and the body weight of the doctor holding me down is too much for me to fight off. I vaguely hear the sucking noises but my brain is in too much fight mode to take in much of what is going on. Then comes the awful feeling of my insides being wrenched out, followed by an explosion of vomit.

'There we go. All over before you knew it. It's only a short time of being uncomfortable,' the doctor says to me. 'You should be grateful we have the technology now to save you and your baby,' he continues. 'Nurse, clean her up and make her comfortable and let her rest.'

After being cleaned up and given some food, I rest. I again sleep well that night and with no bouts of coughing. On waking, the doctor and nurse both walk into my tent.

'Are we ready for your lungs to be drained again?' the doctor asks me.

'No, I feel absolutely fine. I had no coughing last night and I really don't think I need to have it done. I want to leave and go home now please,' I reply.

'No, no, no, you can't go home. You need to stay here and be looked after. We know what is good for you. Now just be still and don't fight it,' he says in a commanding tone, then they both come towards me.

No, this can't keep happening. How the hell am I going to get out of here? I need to get away. Help me somebody, please. Then the whole nightmare begins again.

It is the middle of Winter. Thick snow blankets the streets and all the landscape before you. England in the early 1800s and Christmas is only days away. I have a baby lying in a white cane wicker pram and nowhere to live. I need to find a household that needs some help with cleaning or cooking to earn some money and have a roof over me and my baby's head.

As I amble down the footpath pushing my babe in the pram, I look in each of the windows I pass. Seeing the candlelight flickering to illuminate the rooms and watching the families happy together and nestling around the fireplace glowing with warm red coals and flames keeping them warm and cosy, I yearn to have such love and security that comes with a family. Some of the doors have a Christmas wreath hanging from them and all the houses have a small front yard with a pocket of lawn now covered in deep snow. Fences ranging from wooden pickets to beautiful stone walls secure the houses from the public movement beyond them. The streets and paths are dimly lit by oil lamps lit each night.

One window piques my interest. I peer in and stop to observe for a minute. The dining table is laden with a scrumptious roast lamb and roasted potatoes, pumpkin and peas with a gravy boat filled with rich brown gravy. A candelabra sits in the centre of the table and all the dining setting is placed so precisely. That would be the perfect place to work, I think to myself. Obviously, money is no issue and surely they have servants in a home of that kind.

I bravely push the pram through the gateway and up the small path leading to the front door. I knock loudly and the door soon opens. A woman dressed in a beautiful light-blue, bustled dress appears. 'How can I help you?' she asks me politely.

'I'm looking for work and a place to stay with my baby. I'm very good at house cleaning. I can look after your children, too. I don't mind what I have to do. I will do anything you want me to. I just really need some shelter from this freezing weather for my tiny babe. Please, I'm sure you won't be disappointed with me. I'm a very thorough worker.' I plead.

Looking down into the pram and seeing a tiny little bundle all wrapped in blankets and then up to me, now shivering from the freezing weather, she invites me in.

'Come, we'll talk inside out of this frigid weather,' she says kindly.

The warmth of the fire heated home surrounds my whole being. I feel the cold deep within my bones slowly melt away and a sense of protection and safety fill my body. I take my baby out to hold and comfort her and she gurgles in quiet contentment.

'I don't really need any more help but you can at least stay the night and have some food with us. I will talk to my husband and see what he says about giving you a job.'

'Thank you so much, you are very kind and I am truly grateful' I reply.

'Come and sit down with us, we were just about to eat our evening dinner,' she says as we make our way into the dining room.

The evening is such a delight. Laughter, conversations and smiles shared by all the children and their parents. A true sense of family love is what I am experiencing. After the most soul enriching meal, I am shown to the guest room with a thick, warm duck down patchwork doona laid upon the bed. It was the most beautiful bed I had slept in for a very long time. Cuddling my babe in bed with me, I feel so secure and peaceful, something I haven't felt for a long, long time.

Morning comes too soon after a much-needed peaceful sleep was bestowed upon me. I dress and make my way downstairs and am welcomed by the most appetizing cooked breakfast of bacon and eggs on toast with a pot of tea. I think I am in heaven. The conversation flowed so easily between us all again and I really got on with the children. The husband then told me they would trial me for a week and see how things go. I feel so elated it is hard to constrain myself from bursting out in hugs and kissing them. The beaming smile on my face I'm sure shows them I am overwhelmed by their offer.

It is five days before Christmas and there is a lot of food preparation to be done, along with dressing the children for school and walking them there. I push my baby in the pram when walking the children and do house cleaning through the day. I feel like I am part of their family already and am so happy to be there working and living with them. Life couldn't get any better.

Christmas day arrives and I help prepare the lunch for their friends to come and share. The guests arrive punctually and soon carols are being sung by the fire and everyone is enjoying themselves. Then one of the guests notices a trinket is missing from the mantel piece. The woman of the house comes to look and agrees. Then the guest accuses me of stealing it. I deny it and say I would never do such a thing and why would I ruin such a perfect opportunity like the one I was in now? The guest keeps badgering the woman of the house to act because surely she wouldn't let a thief stay under her own roof.

I am devastated. How can she believe I would do such a thing when I got on so well with the children and them? She knew I was very happy about the situation and she also enjoyed my company but the relentless badgering by the guest is more than she can take and under pressure, she tells me I have to leave.

'Please. You surely don't believe him. He doesn't even know me and how we all get on together. You can't.' I announce in a distressed voice.

'Sorry, Colleen but you must leave now. Go pack your things and go now,' she yells at me, not being able to look me in the eyes while saying it.

I grab my baby and the few things I have and go back downstairs.

Sobbing, I beg, 'Please, where am I going to go? It's Christmas day and nothing is open. It's snowing outside and my baby and I will freeze. Please.'

The woman falters but then the guest opens the door and tells *me to go.*

With tears streaming down my face, I walk out into the blizzard-like weather. Looking back through the window, I can see them all sitting down to eat in the comfort and warmth as I begin to shiver from the icy wind blowing through me.

France in the Renaissance period, when art is a common pastime for many people of the upper classes. Artists are plentiful and beautiful pieces can be found everywhere. Up in an attic of a common building lives one particular artist. She combines her paintings with her spiritual abilities. Some would say it is magic and others, the work of a White Witch. Whatever its nature, the pieces are worthy of being placed in a fine art gallery but nobody is game enough to display them for fear of being connected to the taboo practice of witchcraft. So here, in this little cluttered attic, is this most amazing collection of paintings, collecting dust.

A balding elderly man with grey hair, wearing little round metal spectacles comes knocking on the attic door. The woman opens it and greets the man.

'Can you help me please? I have a very sick boy who needs to get medical help and I can't afford it,' he asks her.

'Come in and we'll talk,' she answers.

Entering the attic and finding two wooden chairs to sit on, the man tells her the story of his demise. She sits and listens about this boy who needs a new heart but travelling abroad was the only option for his survival. It is his son and without her help, he will surely die.

The woman explains there was a way but with no guarantee he will make it to the hospital abroad. She is willing to give it a go if he is.

Without any other options, the man agrees.

She tells him to bring the boy back tomorrow and she will prepare a painting suitable for the job.

Returning the following day with a very ill boy in his arms, she hustles them in.

The boy is about ten years old and very weak indeed. Looking at him, she sits him on one of the wooden chairs.

'Here is the painting I made ready,' she announces.

There before them is a beautiful water-colour painting of a brightly coloured hot air balloon with a wicker basket, a blue sky with a few puffy white clouds and deep green meadows and fields below it. A large oak tree fills the bottom left corner and over the fields is a brown and golden coloured patchwork of crops. In the far distance, in the top right corner of the painting, is a separate piece of land–a country overseas.

'How this works is quite hard to comprehend. I will paint the boy into the wicker basket. As I do, he will physically disappear. Then once I cast the spell over the painting, the hot air balloon will begin its journey abroad, carrying the boy to the hospital that I have encoded into the picture. We can observe his journey through the painting. So if you agree, I can start the process.' she says.

They both nod their heads and watch as she paints the boy into the painting. By the last stroke of the brush the boy went from a fading apparition to vanishing completely.

I know the boy is me in a previous lifetime, because I can completely associate what is happening to him with myself.

I am now floating high in the sky with this magnificent, coloured balloon above me. I lay there limp and weak with the warmth of the hot gas flame keeping me warm as it keeps the aircraft afloat. The striped colours of the balloon are like a rainbow and very calming to watch as it drifts past clouds in the azure sky.

Then as I drift in and out of consciousness, I realise the top half of the balloon and the sky is now in greyscale. The colour is only beneath me and the lower section of the balloon remains without colour. What is happening, I wonder?.

In the attic, as the old man and woman watch the painting, a worried look crosses their faces. 'What's happening?' the man asks, panicked.

'He's getting too weak. The colour is his life force. As he physically weakens the colour fades,' she says despondently. They both sit there, desperately watching and willing the painting to remain coloured.

I don't know what is happening but I am too tired to be worried. I just lay there and continue to watch as the colour comes back for a little while but then fades back into grey.

The last time I open my eyes to see the bright rainbow coloured balloon, it has all faded to grey.

'Mum, the floors look really great,' Mark says to me. 'Come and I'll show you,' 'He takes me by the hand and leads me to the centre of a space-age house. Even though I know it is meant to be my home, it is a very high-tech abode. All white inside with this large dome-shaped Perspex computer. From this, the whole house could be refurbished, redesigned and changed to whatever you wanted it to become. The setting that it was currently on gave the home the wooden vinyl floor covering that I had chosen to go into the house before the transplant. It looks absolutely amazing and I love it. The kitchen is brand new, too and is exactly what I wanted my kitchen to be. I am so happy with the furnishings in my home and really love my floor. The ceiling is extremely high as well, like walking into a large foyer of a grand hotel. Long lights hang from the ceiling and *drop a long way down to become a grand centre piece of the house.*

Mark is so proud showing me the flooring and my new kitchen design. The house also has large floor to ceiling windows opened out to a beautiful grassy outdoor living area. Up-lights are scattered around in the garden and entertaining area, lighting it beautifully. It is my perfect dream home.

My family decide to throw a party for me that night to celebrate having the transplant. All our friends and family come. I am a little overwhelmed by the number of guests we have as a lot of them are my son's friends and all outside dancing and listening to their rap music loudly. I am glad everyone is having a great time but decide to go to bed.

In the morning, when I come back into the centre of my home I am taken aback. Too shocked to comprehend what I am seeing before me; the whole house has changed.

Large glossy white tiles now cover the floor. The kitchen is now blue and completely different to the night before. The grand lights hanging in the centre of the house are gone and purple fluoro tubes illuminate the room. Where has my beautiful home gone? I wonder in despair.

Mark walks into the room and seeing the stunned and disappointed look on my face, he moves to the central dome computer. 'Sorry, Mum. Last night some of the guys wanted to try a different style of house to party in. Don't worry, Mum, I can get your old furnishing back. It's all done by the computer. I just need to go through the settings and get the one you want back.'

I watch him changing the programs and as he does, can't believe what I am seeing before me. The house is in a constant mode of changing floor coverings, kitchen designs and lighting modalities. Even to the point where the outdoor living area changes. One minute a pool is there, then a paved backyard appears. How is this really happen? I have some idea of quantum physics and the different laws of reality but this is way beyond my comprehension.

'How about this one, Mum? This is pretty cool,' Mark asks me.

'No, I just want my wooden vinyl flooring back. The one that I chose and loved.' I frantically reply.

'I'm trying but there are so many combinations to go through,' he answers as I continue to watch the ever-changing house, like looking through a kaleidoscope.

I am now in a state of despair, wondering if I will ever get to live in the house I loved. I just want things to go back to the way they were.

Next thing, it's night-time and Les, Mark, Scott and I are returning home. There had been news of catastrophic earthquakes occurring in the vicinity of where we live.

We know we must get home quickly to check our home is safe and remain there until it's over. It's only five days before Christmas and we had been out shopping together, buying presents for each other.

This is a special Christmas as I'm awaiting a heart transplant. The amount of energy I have left is minimal and I can't walk very far or do anything strenuous.

Opening our front door and turning on the lights, we see our huge Christmas tree that previously stood eight metres high lying across the lounge floor. The dining table and chairs have fallen over and are strewn everywhere. A huge five-centimetre crack splits our main wall in half. We go into the kitchen where smashed crockery and glass cover the floor. Staying out of the area to not get any glass in our shoes and feet, we stand there taking in the sight of our shattered home and look at each other in despair. Then came another tremor. The floor shakes and the chandelier lights begin swaying violently. A crescendo of smashing glass along with the *rumbling sound of the earth beneath us deafens our ears. Losing our balance as the floor begins to split, we all jump to the same side of the crack to remain together. Holding hands in an attempt to make us feel safe, we watch as the crack becomes a ravine.*

Now seeing the ramifications of the earth's violent rumbling, one half of our house is now on a lower level. This means we can no longer get out through our front door. If we stay here, only God knows what the outcome would be. Our only option is the ceiling. The centre of our house has a large glass dome to let in the natural light, now shattered into a million pieces all over the floor. We just have to work out how to get up there because our ceiling is very high.

Surveying what was left in our home, Les comes up with the idea of dragging the Christmas tree over and standing it up. Hopefully then it may come close to reaching the broken hole in the ceiling and we can climb out. The boys help their dad pull the tree over from where it lay, and with much effort, they manage to get it upright. With the higher ceiling however, it isn't tall enough to reach the top.

All of us are looking at the distance between the top of the tree and the ceiling, the cogs in our heads turning frantically. Mark suddenly gets up and goes over to retrieve a chair. Climbing the tree while holding on to it, Scott and Les then follow suite. I also grab a chair and begin to climb. It takes some time to make the chairs and other items stable enough to climb but they eventually succeed. The escape route out of here is now suitable enough to be used.

Les leads the way climbing up the huge Christmas tree. Scott follows, then Mark begins to climb. Les finally makes it to the ceiling and with a final heave, pulls himself up through the roof top. He is now on the outside of the building. He sticks his head through telling Scott where to move next as the whole structure isn't stable. Mark is about halfway up the tree when I begin my ascent.

I am tired and short of breath after helping to get the escape structure built. I start my climb but find it very difficult. Looking up and seeing Les and Scott on the outside of the roof, I am glad that it is working and Mark is almost out but don't have it in me to go on any further.

Mark turns around and looks down at me, saying, 'Come on Mum. You can do it; I'll wait for you.'

'No, you keep going. I'll be there soon.'

Mark continues climbing and is nearly at the top. Looking down again, he says, 'Come on Mum, you can make it.'

'I can't, I'm too tired and weak. You need to go on without me and get to safety,' *I reply in an assertive manner.*

Les yells out, 'Come on dear, we'll wait for you. You can make it.'

Mark looks down at me with distress etched in frown lines on his face and once again says, 'Please Mum, you can do it. I'm not leaving you here.'

Then comes another tremor and the ground and tree begin to shake.

'Go on now, Mark. You have to get to safety before it's too late,' *I beg.*

'Come on Mark, you need to get up here with us now,' *shouts Les.*

Looking up and seeing the three faces of my family looking down through the hole, I am relieved that they at least will be safe, Les will look after them.

'Come on dear, keep climbing. We'll be here to help you out,' *Les says.*

'No, I can't. I'm too tired, I haven't got it in me to fight anymore,' *I reply, defeated.*

With another tremor in the ground, Les gives me a sorrowful look as I stare up from the base of the huge Christmas tree.

Walking past a television shop window, I notice people starting to gather around a 60s-style black and white TV, the shop fronts also of that era. They are watching the news, an announcement by NASA. The reporter states that NASA have made a catastrophic mistake in their calculations. The world, which was to be ending in 25 years, is now having its doomsday in two and a half weeks. Shock and panic grip them. Screaming, yelling and people running in the streets in all directions. No one knows what to do. What is the escape plan? Hell. How are we going to get off this planet?

As I run home to tell Les, a woman grabs me and pulls me to the side. 'Don't worry, I'm not going to hurt you. I have a way of surviving if you're interested?' the woman says to me in a sincere tone.

Without having any other plan, I decide to take a chance on her. 'OK,' I reply.

She grabs my hand and leads me to a doorway in a darkened building on one of the side streets. We enter the building and she turns on the lights.

'In here,' she motions to me with a nod of her head.

I obediently follow her into a huge warehouse. In the centre of the room is a giant blow-up igloo. It is white and stands about three metres high. There is a flap held in place with Velcro. She leads me inside and contains all the basic necessities for living: A compact kitchen, bed, small table, chairs for two people and a two-seater sofa. I am still trying to figure out how it is going to save me and Les. If the world is going to explode from a meteorite strike, then this isn't going to be much help.

'This igloo is made from a very special material. It can withstand atomic-level force. It has its own recycling system to supply fresh

air and a crystal powered generator to keep enough electricity running to power lights and the kitchen stove. However, the main machine that keeps the igloo inflated is a very old-fashioned clockwork mechanism. I'm sure your husband would be able to fix it if it broke down. A simple tool kit is all that's required to maintain the mechanism. Come and have a look at it,' she proudly tells me.

As I see the mechanism, I am impressed by the ingenuity of it. Here was this little mechanical man wearing brown trousers and a white buttoned up shirt. A boater hat rests on his head. He has tiny leather shoes attached to the pedals. He sits on a miniature Penny Farthing bicycle with the wheels attached to the cogs in the machine. As he pedals, the cogs and their interlinking teeth wind many integrated and various sized cogs. It is truly impressive; a bizarre combination of futuristic technology powered by old-fashioned engineering. A true marriage of past supporting the future.

'Here is the tool kit that has the instruments and tools to repair the mechanisms,' the woman says as she hands over a small black leather kit.

As I peer inside it, she says, 'Your husband is quite capable of being able to repair this machine. He was a television repair man before and he has a scientific mind. He can always seem to engineer something to keep it working.' I look at her in genuine gratitude and as our eyes meet, staring into each other's souls for a split second, she says, 'Just remember, if the mechanism stops then the life support igloo will begin to collapse. No air will be produced and once it fully collapses, then you will die.'

After going home to Les and telling him of the events that had taken place that evening, we agree it is the best option to go with. The following day, we go to the shops and get our survival stores and equipment, then find the woman and pick up the large box containing the igloo. Having decided the previous evening on best place to go and set up our igloo, we drive out into the countryside and deep within the forest, isolated from the main population. We think it is the safest option.

We assemble the igloo and the machine blows it up in no time at all. The furniture and all our things are now in place. It isn't quite what we are used but it is home.

Days pass without much event, then I notice the ceiling falling slowly down towards me. 'Les, you need to fix the little man. He's stopped working and the igloo is falling,' I say with urgency. He immediately retrieves his tool kit and proceeds to fix the mechanical man. After using some screwdrivers and other instruments, the little man begins to pedal and the roof rises again. I am so relieved.

A few more days pass when I notice the ceiling falling again.

'Les, it's happening again,' I tell him.

He rambles through the tool kit trying different screwdrivers but none seem to do the job. Watching the ceiling falling closer and with him not being able to get the mechanical man working, I begin to panic.

'Hurry. You have to fix it,' I shout at him.

'None of the tools are doing it. I need a different one. I'm going to have to drive back into town and get one,' he replies in a state of stress.

'How much time will you need? I don't know how long this igloo has before it completely collapses.'

'I'll be as quick as I can. Don't worry, I'll be back before you know it. I won't let anything happen to you, darling.'

Time comes to a standstill. Eternity passes as I watch the falling ceiling. I am fixated by the thought of how long it might be until my life support failed, overwhelmed by the white expanse closing in on me.

'I'm back darling. Don't worry, I'll soon have it all working again.'

I Can See Clearly Now

Les's voice echoes through the failing tent.

Watching him frantically working on the machine, all my hopes ride on him saving us. Then the much-awaited site of the white expanse retreating comes as a blessing.

'There we go dear. I told you I wouldn't let anything happen to you,' he says.

I toss him the most grateful smile and feel so blessed to have him with me.

Once again, many days pass without any events. Life is hopeful and I feel safe with Les here by my side. One night, I awake with the sense of not being able to breathe properly.

'Les, I think the life support is failing again,' I say, shaking him to wake up.

He stands up but the ceiling is already only just above his head. There isn't enough power to turn on the lights, so he has to scramble around in the dark to find his tool kit. A stifling, oppressive feeling cloaks me as Les flails around in the darkness.

I can't move and my airways are struggling to work properly. I am beginning to gasp for air and can hear Les rapidly tinkering in his effort to repair the mechanical man.

'Nothing seems to be working, darling. None of the tools are doing the job. I'm trying my best. I'm so sorry dear. I love you,' he says in a teary voice.

As Les and I exit our space shuttle, we walk down the stairs onto a planet somewhere out in our galaxy. NASA had sent people to various planets for survival, intending that once earth is inhabitable again we can all go home We'd all been given a manual on the inhabitants of each of the planets we landed on. It briefed us on the rituals and customs performed, along with the laws of nature and survival skills needed there.

The planet we are on is a plant-based lifeform but the living environment is inside the crust. There are large openings on the surface that lead down to it. We peruse the desolate landscape before us. Nothing but grey, dead rocky surface extends for miles. Les and I look at each other, hold hands and begin to walk.

After a short while, we come across a tunnel opening. With a glance of approval to each other, we enter the hole. Tall enough for us to stand up in and wide enough for us to walk side-by-side. It is a gentle enough gradient to be able to walk down quite comfortably. The darkness soon looms all around as we continue to move further below the surface crust. Then a small light filters up towards us.

Before our eyes is a cavernous area from which a beautiful, intense light shines. Vegetation surrounds us. Magnificent green plants, some with the most brilliantly coloured flowers, and vines hanging from the ceiling. They seem to communicate with each other. We both stand there in amazement watching the rhythmic kaleidoscope of colours and greenery swaying and turning toward each other.

We continue further down into the cavern feeling no threat at all. A large reservoir of water fills the central floor. We decide to set up camp in a small clearing not too far from the water. We don't want to go anywhere near the plants until we are more familiar with our surroundings.

Over the next few days, Les and I explore the unfamiliar territory we are now living in. Reading the manuals and learning the customs, we eventually start to feel at home. We learn which plants we could use for food and how we can start to grow our own seedlings from earth. Except for being isolated from any other civilization, we are very happy. Our seedlings grow into beautiful vegetables and being surrounded by the calming rhythm of the plant life forms before us is just magical.

Les comes walking back towards me after going on one of his explorations. With an excited expression on his face, he hands me a most unusual plant.

'Look what I found darling. It is the most beautiful plant I've ever seen. I thought you may like it,' he eagerly says as he hands me the gorgeous flower.

Taking a closer look at it, I ask, 'Where did you find it?'

'Just beyond the outer walls of this cavern. It was there all by itself in the dark,' he replies.

Frantically looking through the manual, I find the information on the flower. It is the life force that gives the plants light. Without this master plant nothing can survive.

'Didn't you read this manual?' I ask, distressed.

'No. I thought you were doing the research and would tell me anything I needed to know,' he responds.

'Well this is the life force of this planet. We can't survive here without it,' I reply angrily.

Les, looking at me in absolute remorse and despair says, 'I'm so sorry darling. I didn't know.'

Before our eyes, the plants all droop and wither. The light that once brightly illuminated the cavern is rapidly dimming. Les and I just look into each other's eyes as everything around goes into total darkness.

Les and I somehow manage to land on another planet. I don't know how we got here but this planet surface is nothing but rocks and boulders. There isn't much light, either. It's like being in a dark grey cloud-filled sky at sunset. Things are visible but only just. I don't have a manual for this planet, which means we will have to stay hidden and try and observe the rituals of this seemingly God-forsaken land.

As we make our way across the rocky terrain, neither Les nor I *are feeling very hopeful. What could ever live and survive on this lifeless surface? There doesn't seem to be movement of any kind, not even a breeze. No vegetation or life of any sort. Nothing.*

After walking for quite some time, we decide to take cover for the night, even though we have no idea of the time or if it has got dark. We settle in amongst some boulders that have a small patch of smooth dirt to lay on. We sit together for a while without saying anything. I think neither of us knows what to expect from this hostile environment. Then in the distance, I see something moving. I nudge Les and point in the direction I was looking. Both of us strain our eyes in the dim light to see what it is. Then more movement. Around us, the rocks begin to rumble and vibrate. Les and I quickly jump up and run further away from the rocks.

Rocks and boulders are rolling in chaotic directions. Then, unbelievably, the rocks all start to stack up on top of each other and transform into giant rock men. How can this be? That's not possible. Now towering around us are these giant rock beings that all begin to move.

Ogling in astonishment, we both observe the gathering and moving of these unusual life forms. Some seem to gather together as if they are a family, while others just roam around, occasionally bending down to pick up and eat smaller pebbles. More rock beings come into this area. What is going to happen?

Thump, thump reverberates through the land. Two rock men came into view. The others seem to welcome the newcomers. We watch as they seem to harmoniously wander around together. Three thumps are then felt. In the distance, another large rock being comes into view. As the newcomer comes closer, the largest of the rock clan stomps over towards him, the ground really rumbling and shaking. The sound is like a clash of the Titans. Loud, thunderous booms echoing through the still air, shaking your inner being. The roaring sound of rocks crashing and tumbling carries on for ages until only the rock man of this clan remains standing.

Watching the continuing interactions of these beings is fascinating. It is if they are sentient and can communicate. They also appear to have some kind of hierarchy. The big one of this clan, the one that fought the intruder, seems to be the leader. They continue to slowly stroll amongst each other and enjoy their social interactions.

Luckily, none of them spot Les and I still crouching low away from the main group. Two thumps are felt again followed by a group of them congregating closer to where the thumps came from. This must be the way they communicate, through vibration. Maybe they can't see Les and I. We can most probably move around them without even being noticed. At least it was some hope.

Les and I eventually fall asleep while still trying to watch them. It had been a very long and stressful day. Waking in the morning, Les and I only see all the loose rocks scattered around the landscape. No giant beings were anywhere to be found. Curiously looking at each other, we both stand up and walk amongst the rocks.

The day doesn't differ much from the night, so Les and I don't really know which is which. I guess it doesn't really matter, we are living in a totally different world now. No longer on Earth and bound by our society's need to be ruled and regulated by time. Here, time is definitely not of the essence.

Each day we observe the rituals and sequences of thumps which seem to make a code. One thump means it is time to rest. Two thumps are an invitation to come over and socialize. Three thumps are an aggressive call, there's a fight to be had. They seem to be a culture of primitive lifeforms. They grow by rubbing pebbles onto themselves, which are then absorbed into their system. Their rock bodies grow like ours.

It feels like Les and I have been here forever. Each day we live in a state of constant fear, not knowing when a rock being may come our way and destroy us. We have to tread carefully amongst them to gather grasses and any edible food. This is treacherous. One step from these gargantuan beings means instant death. Just the mere roaming of them is dangerous enough, we don't want to do anything to set them off in our direction.

We build ourselves a house made from rocks that never seem to morph into a being.

One day, Les returns from gathering some food. Pleased by his haul, he excitedly jumps three times outside our house. Entering to give me the supplies he'd gathered, we both feel the rumblings. We look at each other in surprise. It is way too early for them to get up. Why is this happening now?

'What did you just do?' I ask Les.

'Nothing,' he responds.

'How many jumps did you just do outside the house?' I demand.

'I did three. Why?'

'No. Three is the fight call. They've seen you as a threat now and will come over and destroy our house and us,' I yell.

The blood drains from Les's face, shocked by the mortal mistake he has just made. Thunderous noise and earthquake-like vibrations are felt as the rock beings head over in our direction. We stand there and stare into each other's horrified eyes.

Pitch black surrounds us except for the brilliant white stars speckling the blank canvas. Standing on this large, flat rectangular rock floating deep in outer space, Les and I have somehow been placed here. The rock is about two-and-a-half kilometres long and one-and-a-half kilometres wide. The depth is 20 metres. Along the side is a name in large Roman lettering: EXODUS.

Far, far away in the unreachable distance, we can see our planet Earth. Vaguely making out some of the blue patches on it, we realise the planet hasn't completely died yet. Somehow Les intuitively knows our mission here is the survival of our planet. While we are alive here on Exodus, then there is hope for humankind. I am extremely weak now and don't have much left in me at all. Les tells me to sit where I am while he scouts the surface to see what there is for us to survive.

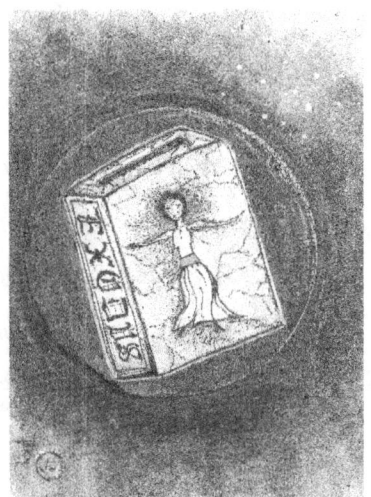

Lying down as I am too tired to sit up, I slowly drift into a slumber, the still darkness blanketing me. Woken by Les shaking me, I sit up and listen to his findings.

He explains that on the other side of Exodus there is a nearby rock we can jump onto. He thinks this rock looks like it has some vegetation that may be edible but didn't know what else was on there. He wants me to come with him to explore this other rock. Seeing how eager he is about this expedition, I agree to go with him.

After making our way to the other side of Exodus, I see how wide the gap to jump to the other rock is. Down the side of Exodus is nothing but a perpetual drop into the abyss. If I can't make the jump then it is all over. Looking at each other, Les lets go of my hand and runs full speed to the edge of Exodus. Holding my breath as I watch him take a mighty leap, I want to close my eyes in case he doesn't make it but I can't. Thankfully, my eyes bless me with the vision of him landing on to the rock in a crouched position. I let out my breath and sigh with relief.

Shit. It's my turn now. I know Les did it first, so it can be done but I am very weak and doubt my energy level. Les nodded and smiled across at me, so I know I have to try. I charge towards the edge of Exodus, my legs moving as fast as they can. Without thinking, I leap into the mouth of the abyss.

'You made it, dear. I knew you could,' was what I hear Les telling me.

I made it. I didn't think I was going to.

Les helps me get up from the ground where I landed with a thud. I wasn't really hurt, just shaken up. We explore the area around us and discover that in the rocky outcrops and small caves there is a wide variety of vegetation. We pick and taste many before choosing which ones we preferred the taste of. After gathering a small handful that we can fit into our clothing, we make our way back.

Looming before us is the dreaded jump across the abyss. I made the leap before but my energy is now more depleted. I suggest to Les we just stay on the rock for the night and return in the morning. He explains he remembered something about dangerous creatures hunting at night and it may not be safe. So, after watching Les run and take his jump and landing safely, I know it is my turn. Too tired to really fear the jump, I muster up as much energy as I can and run toward the edge. Pushing off with all my might, I leap high and just focus on Les waiting on the other side for me. Landing with a thump, I am so relieved to feel the ground beneath my feet. Picking myself up from the ground, I stand up and tearfully look at Les. We slowly journey back to our home base.

I don't know how many days we'd been on Exodus when Les decided to take the journey to the rock to get food by himself. He knows I am too weak to keep making the trek, so I stay behind and wait for him to return. On returning one time, Les finds me lying down flat on my back, eyes closed.

'Wake up Colleen,' he says, shaking me gently.

'No, I'm too tired,' is my weak response.

'You have to sit up. You can't stay lying down. Life on Earth is depending on you for survival.'

'I don't care, I can't do it anymore,' I say with utter dejection.

'Come on darling, you can do it. Please,' he pleas.

'I don't care if all the lights go out in the universe. I haven't got anything left in me,' I whisper. Then laying there stretched out on Exodus, I begin to feel cold. Slowly, all the stars go out and our blue distant home planet slowly turns dark, leaving me blanketed in a black void.

What I have found interesting about this nightmare, is the conversations, words, sounds and actions happening around me and to me over those four days, were absorbed into the reality of my living nightmare, just as the plasmapheresis procedure was. I had that procedure seven times between day-1 and day-11 post-surgery, no wonder it was on my mind.

It is said, hearing is the last of the senses to go before death and I can only conclude I heard and felt things that were happening around me and these elements were absorbed into my brain and formed my four-day nightmare.

Looking objectively at some of the themes of the nightmare, I wonder if some of my very deepest fears were given wings there?

By far the biggest theme was one of helplessness in the face of authority. For a large part of the nightmare, I was trapped in some kind of dystopian authoritarian regime where everything I said was not believed. People of trust, doctors and nurses, accusing me of conspiracy, administering mind altering drugs against my will, persistently working to make me admit my role in a conspiracy of which I knew nothing.

The most bizarre chapter of that four-day nightmare was me and Les surviving on desolate planets.

People and things from my life made guest appearances. A meteor careering towards earth saw Les and me take shelter in a blow-up igloo. Was this the igloo from my childhood which covered the pool in Winter?

In the nightmare the boys and my brothers took drugs, which upset me and had me feeling helpless. Did the drug taking by my brothers in my youth disturb me at a level so deep that it took this nightmare to have my fears and the trauma of this period of our lives manifest?

Aside from the theme of helplessness, another recurring theme was me striving to survive and eventually choosing to give up but with Les and the boys pleading with me not to die.

I didn't die. I survived.

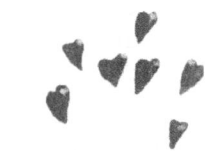

I'm Still Standing
– Elton John

The final instalment of my four-day nightmare happened when, despite my heart not starting independently, the decision was made to stitch me up and bring me out of the induced coma. Obviously, this was touch and go.

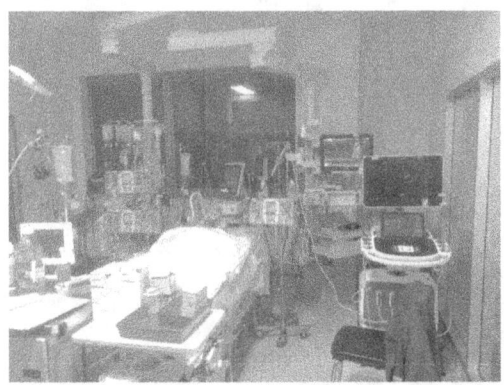

I had lost a huge amount of blood over a long period of time and had gone through the State's supply of my blood type, with additional blood flown in from South Australia. The doctors had told Les and the boys that closing me up had nothing to do with me 'being out of the woods' and there was still a very real chance I wouldn't make it; the heart still wasn't working very well.

The decision to bring me out of the coma coincided with Les and I being on a planet called Exodus during the nightmare and had clear parallels to my precarious physical state and Les begging me to stay with him.

'Do you know where you are Colleen?' asked an English nurse. 'I'm at Fiona

Stanley Hospital,' I answered.

'Do you know what you have had done?' she asked.

'A heart transplant.'

'Do you know who the Prime Minister is?' she asked next.

Not ever being one for following politics or taking much notice of things like that, I was racking my brain. Eventually I came up with, 'I know the American President is Trump.'

'That's good enough for me,' she jokingly said. 'What year is it?' was the next game item from the nurse.

'It's 2016,' I quickly answered.

'No, it's 2017,' she stated firmly.

Hearing this, my brain went into overload, scrambling through the events that had happened. Scott's graduation, Christmas at home in the pool having water gun fights. No, that can't be right.

'What year is it?' came the pick-a-box question again from the nurse.

'2016,' I instinctively replied.

'No, it's 2017,' came the same firm answer.

That can't be right, I thought. That means Scott would have to do all his driving lessons and apply for his driver's licence all over again. No, what's going on, my scrambled brain was trying to figure out.

'What year is it?' came the same question.

Feeling quite distressed by what this meant according to my memory, I abruptly replied, 'I know you say it's 2017 but I still think it's 2016.'

I seemed to drift in and out of a dream state once again.

Memories of the failing igloo from my nightmare and waving blackness before my eyes kept coming into my focus. Night came and was a restless and stressful experience. I had to wear a heavy respirator that expressed warm moist oxygen to help support my lungs. I kept on wanting to pull it off and my weird dreams floated in and out of my mind all night. I couldn't make out my room but could hear the different noises. There was a sound like lollies being dropped into a container. I was getting annoyed by the nurse thinking she was eating lollies on her night shift. It was rude to eat while she was meant to be a professional looking after me, not eating lollies. I found out about four days later the noise was medication tablets for the dialysis. It's funny how things sound like something else when you can't see what's going on.

Morning didn't come quick enough after a long restless night. A group of doctors came around. One of them was Dr A because I knew his voice. After the preliminary test of pushing and squeezing their hands, they asked if I was in any pain.

I responded, 'No, but I can't see.' All I can make out are waving black walls around me and bits of light and bright colour on my right side.

'What do you mean, you can't see?' asked Dr A.

'I can't see,' I repeated.

'Can you see this?' Dr A asked.

Not being able to see what he was asking me to see, I said, 'No.'

He came close to my right side near my head and he asked, 'Can you see this?' He was holding something bright red but I didn't know what it was.

'I can see red,' I answered, straining my eyes.

'It's my stethoscope,' he told me.

'You're wearing a blue shirt.'

'Good, you can see something then,' came his relieved response.

'Can you see me?' asked a female doctor who was on my left side.

Turning in the direction of her voice, I said, 'No.'

Low murmuring proceeded between them, then Dr A asked, 'Tell me when you see this.'

Eventually, I saw a bright hot pink thing.

'I see pink,' I answered. It turned out to be a bright pink teddy with a silver tiara named 'Princess'. My dear friend Amanda had bought it in, being as 'Princess' was my alias.

'You have been asleep for quite a long time. It may take a while for your brain to wake up properly. We'll check on it again tomorrow.' Dr A told me.

I never saw them leave but could hear them go.

Les, Scott, Mark, Mum, Hon and Eddie came in to see me. Only two at a time were allowed, so the others had to sit in the waiting room and take it in turns. I was finding it hard to keep my eyes open but they kept talking and I answered back when needed. It was so nice having them with me again. It took me quite some time to grasp the reality that they weren't all dead, my nightmare still felt very real.

Mum was always at the hospital along with my brother Eddie. Mum filled me in on what had happened after the transplant. When the new heart was put in, it wouldn't start up. A 'stunned heart' is what they call it. Sometimes it takes up to eight hours before they can close you up in surgery, however, my heart showed no sign of wanting to work at all. With my chest still cracked open and attached to an Extracorporeal Membrane Oxygenation machine (ECMO machine), I was brought up to the ICU.

For the first two days, I had two nurses in with me at all times. One was there to watch the ECMO and the other for the other machines. I had 14 machines and monitors on me. The ECMO was what had kept me alive for the first four days. The machine does all the functioning of the heart and lungs. You can have an empty chest cavity and the ECMO can keep you alive by oxygenating the blood and pumping it around to all the other organs of the body. As I've mentioned, the decision to stich me up was made after four days in this state, with my new heart just showing signs of starting.

When I saw Scott, I asked him, 'How is your hand?'

He said, 'It's fine Mum.'

Remembering the nightmare, I knew he had come off his bike and broken it.

Puzzled, I asked, 'Do you still have your car?'

'Yes Mum,' was his reply.

'Did you buy a motorbike?' my inquiry continued. My brain, trying to get the truth out of him.

'No Mum,' was his short, puzzled response.

'Didn't you come off your bike and break your hand?' I asked.

'Oh no, that was Frank. He came off and broke it. He's alright though, just got his hand in a plaster and did a bit of damage to his bike.'

'Oh. I thought it was you and that you had sold your car,' was my relieved response.

In my nightmare state before regaining consciousness, I could obviously hear what was being talked about around my bed. It went in and for whatever reason, the words, phrases and situations were woven into my nightmare.

I can't remember who came in with whom, my brain was pretty foggy. I remember when Eddie came in, I could just make him out in his bright yellow safety work shirt.

'Hi Sis,' he excitedly said, glad to see me alive and awake.

Remembering the nightmare and all his bad behaviour, I brazenly asked, 'You're not on drugs, are you?'

'No Sis,' he laughed.

'You sure?' At this stage, my nightmare was still very real and as far as I knew, Eddie was, apart from a murderer, a drug taking thug.

'Sis, I haven't done drugs for a long time,' he happily answered going along with my delirious state.

When Mark came in, he told me the flooring looked really great. I told him I remembered him coming in and telling me. He looked a bit surprised and said he had told me when he visited me while in the coma and asked if I wanted to listen to some music on Spotify. My response was quite a shock to him when I said I didn't want the phone anywhere near me and not to play the Spotify playlist. He said I was quite distressed, trying to push the phone away when he went to play it just after I came out of the coma. Still not sure of what reality I had been in, I just told him it was all part of a nightmare I had been in.

Again, things said around my bed and said to me were absorbed into my nightmare but distorted to an incredible degree.

Les was just so glad to see me alive. Holding my hand in sheer relief, words were hard to find and I had no idea how long I had been asleep or the events that had unfolded over the previous four days. Not only had I been in a nightmare but so had all my family and friends.

Les and the boys and the whole family had been dealing with the very real prospect I wasn't going to make it.

The day after waking, the surgeon, Mr C, came in to see me. Having not met him before, I asked how it all went, not realising all the events that had occurred.

The only words he could say were, 'That is one night I never want to remember.'

I could feel his immense distress and felt really sorry for him.

The days were a blur as I slowly began to recover. I was still attached to machines because my new heart wasn't working properly yet, still on dialysis for my kidneys and had an arterial line in one arm and a PICC line in the other. Both these lines went directly into the heart. The main machine did most of the work to support the new heart in getting the blood pumping around my body. They could tell how much work my heart was doing and how much the machine was needed for support. I still had to lay flat because as soon as the bed was tilted, my blood pressure would go up. It wasn't yet strong enough to pump upwards.

It was Monday, the second day of waking up. The doctors asked about my vision but nothing had changed. The vision tests were done again and more low murmuring was heard. They said it may take a while for my brain to wake up but things were slowly heading in the right direction with my heart.

Mum told me that Will had been brought into the hospital the second day after my surgery. He had a head injury and was on another ward. She went on to tell me that Geoff had been flown in from the mine up north, having had a stroke. So, between her and Eddie, they did the rounds visiting the three of us.

It then made sense to me. When Will was admitted he entered my nightmare, obviously hearing the conversation while in my coma; Geoff also entered.

Gradually I was piecing together the connections between events in my nightmare with events and conversations taking place around me. I asked Mum if there had been a 40-degree day? She told me there was a stinker of a day when they came into visit. Yes, another correlation between the nightmare and reality. I hadn't revealed any of it to anyone yet. I was still too weak to talk much.

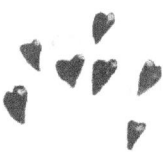

Breathe
– Pink Floyd

During my time in ICU, Eddie had driven up to where my dad lives in Wongan Hills, a wheatbelt farming town 180 kms from Perth. He went there to pick him up and bring him down to see me. When Dad came into the ICU and saw me with all the machines attached, he turned around and sat in the waiting room. He was too distressed to see me in that state and was finding it hard to cope. At 88 years of age, to see his baby daughter like that was not what he could deal with. He wanted to go back to Wongan the next day and asked Eddie to keep him informed. Poor Dad, I can't imagine how stressful it must have been to see me like that. Eddie would regularly take photos of me once I was awake to show Dad how well I was going. He would phone him and let him talk to me once I was on the up, just to let him know things were going in the right direction. Dad was devastated again when Eddie told him I was blind. Poor Dad, is all I can say.

Hon came in each day. She had the stressful job of keeping most of my friends up to date with what had been going on with me. Mum kept the rest of the family informed. Hon was with me when I heard the South African nurse come over from another patient and say, 'Oh, it's so good to see you awake Colleen.' That nurse (or her voice) played a significant part in my nightmare as an evil, sadistic protagonist. On hearing her voice, the nightmare and all the horrific things she had done to me, welled up and in a venomous voice I said, 'No, not YOU.'

Shocked by my response she just said, 'That's OK, I'll catch you a bit later.'

Hon was taken aback by my vicious response. She could see I was stressed by the appearance of this nurse and she calmly said, 'No Hon, she was one of the nurses that was so protective and cared for you so well. She was such a wonderful and caring nurse.'

'Well she was the one torturing me and wanting to kill me in my nightmare,' I answered. Then I felt bad about my response and apologised to her when I saw her again.

Hon told me how she had to show a photo of me to the two nurses who looked after me in the first two days. I had blown up so much they couldn't even open my eye lids to put in the drops. I was a Michelin man beyond recognition. When she showed them a photo that was only taken three weeks before, the nurses said they were quite surprised I looked so well. She told them this is the person they were fighting for.

Hon told me how she would do her crossword puzzles and ask me questions. After getting no response, she would say, 'Well you're not much good at crosswords are you, chipmunk cheeks.' She said the nurses found that very amusing. She told them I wouldn't be offended and would see the funny side of it. It was Hon's way of coping, seeing me as I was. As she said, 'What else do you do? Sit there in worry and fear or try and make it more tolerable to cope with?'

This was especially so when on the very first day, the doctors told everyone there was nothing more they could do. They had put everything they could in and on me. It was now up to me to pull through.

Hon said that's when she knew things were really bad. There was no more backup plan. I already had every possible machine-aid attached.

The morning after the transplant, Hon was the first person to see me on her way to work as Les had rung her to tell her the doctor had phoned around midnight and told him things hadn't gone to plan and to expect the worse. Hon told me she walked into my room and turned straight around and had to go back outside and collect herself. To walk in and see all the monitors and machines, with two nurses attending was beyond her comprehension. As she was leaving to tell her work she wouldn't be coming in for the day, she saw Les and the boys arriving. All she could say to Les was, 'Prepare yourself.'

I can't imagine how stressful it must have been for everyone who loved me so deeply to see me in that situation. Especially the boys, they were a lot younger and with no experience of things like that. Even Hon told me she thought she was pretty good with medical things but nothing prepared her for this.

I told Hon about my nightmare and how in part of it, she would be there stroking my head and hair and how comforting it was. She confirmed it was exactly what she used to do while playing the 'feeling swanky' playlist. Amazing how pieces of the nightmare-reality jigsaw puzzle began to fit together.

On Tuesday morning, now one week from surgery, the ophthalmologist came in to see me. He did his test and looked into my eyes with his light. Mum was there when I was having this done. He told me he was pretty sure it was permanent. He would come back next week and check again but not to get my hopes up. He had seen it before when people had lost a lot of blood. It's from a lack of oxygen to the optic nerve which tells the brain how to see. It's funny really, I never felt upset or worried about being blind or the thought of not seeing again. Whether I was still too weak from the surgery or because I have always taken everything that happens to me in my stride, I really don't know but I never got angry or stressed about it.

The nights were long, I never slept. Frequently throughout the night, I would ask the nurse what the time was. I would lie there designing my new kitchen and how I would decorate it, right down to the finest details. By the third day, I told the doctors I wasn't sleeping at all. They explained it was very common because of the large quantity of steroids needed to prevent rejection. They prescribed some sleeping tablets and that night I slept much better.

The heart still wasn't working very well by itself yet and so I still had to remain quite flat in bed and needed help to turn over on my side. Bed baths were done so nicely. It felt very soothing and comforting to have your body wiped and gently cleaned. I especially loved it when they washed my hair in the cap, then massaged my head. It just made me feel fresh and human again.

When Les and the boys came in to visit after the ophthalmologist had been, the doctors told them the news. I didn't know until sometime after that when Les learned of my blindness it had been another roller coaster ride for them all, just as they were allowing themselves to feel relief about me still being alive. Now they had the devastating news I would most probably be blind. How was life going to be with a blind wife and mother to look after? Would Les have to give up work to look after me? How was I going to do things, especially being diabetic and having to take insulin shots five times a day? I wouldn't be able to drive and all the things we take for granted would now be very tricky tasks to overcome and manage.

All these thoughts were running through Les's head for quite a few days. The boys were thinking, how was I going to do all the things I used to love doing before the transplant? It would be a huge adjustment for all of us to deal with. They never showed me they were worried and were all still so glad I was alive.

Stephen had been in most days to visit through this whole ordeal. He was, however, in a rehab centre for around three months at this stage, so his councillor would drive him and be there for support. He never dreamed I would be needing a heart transplant. It was a regular event for me to go in and have stents put in and I had never made an issue of the state of my failing heart. Life always returned to normal as soon as I was home from hospital. As I've mentioned, I never was the type to make a problem out of any health issues I was going through. I protected the family from all the worry and possible outcomes simply because I didn't want to stress them. Stephen took it extremely hard seeing me in that state, then finding out I was blind was something that I think to this very day, he finds hard to accept.

In the second week, fluid started building up around the heart wall. They needed to release the fluid but didn't really want to put me under another general anaesthetic, so they asked if I would do it under a local? I agreed, not knowing what I was in for.

I have a pretty high pain threshold but this was not pleasant at all. I kept wincing as the knife dug around between my ribs trying to find the right spot and complained it was hurting.

'Give her some more Ventolin,' was the order.

In my mind, I remembered the doctors had said I had a very unusual response to Ventolin. It was like an allergic reaction that affected my lungs in a bad way. They had never come across anyone allergic to Ventolin before.

The pain still high, more Ventolin was given. My mind was going into panic but I was getting drowsy and my lungs were starting to rattle, then there was nothing...

'How long has she been asleep?' I heard a doctor ask.

'A few hours now,' the nurse answered.

'How much Ventolin has she had?' Then very assertively, he said, 'You need to wake her up now. She can't have Ventolin. Wake her up.'

I could vaguely hear this conversation and then the nurse gently shaking me and trying to wake me up but all I wanted to do was go back to sleep. She had my dinner there and was cutting it up and trying to feed me to help get me awake. The last thing I wanted was to have food shoved in my mouth but I managed to swallow a few mouthfuls.

It turns out that being given Ventolin when I have an adverse reaction to this drug was a case of miscommunication, or should I say, lack of communication between the Transplant and ICU teams. No one's fault exactly but a good example of how complex my treatment was at this critical time. There was no lasting damage but it was certainly one experience I never wanted to go through again.

I spent exactly two weeks in the ICU and during the last week they did a CAT scan on my head to see if a stroke may have caused the vision issue. They were looking for answers. I was the first person this had happened to and they were trying to work out why. No signs of a stroke or brain trauma were found.

The last three days in ICU, I had come off dialysis and my heart was working by itself. I managed to sit up in bed with the help of the physiotherapist but only for short periods, my blood pressure would still go up with the strain on the heart having to pump harder in an upright position. My heart rate was also an issue.

My resting heart rate was 120 bpm. This is normal and nothing to worry about. When you are given a new heart, the vagus nerve is cut. It regulates the heart rate but with no control centre, the new heart keeps beating quite fast because 'the *fat controller* has left the station'; for those of you who don't know, he was in 'Thomas the Tank Engine'!

In layman's terms, one of the jobs of the vagus nerve is to stimulate muscles in the heart, where it helps to lower the resting heart rate but because I didn't have that, my heart had to wait until hormones in the blood stream kicked in. They would give my heart the signal to work harder if my muscles needed more blood under new stress, such as exercise. So, without the vagus nerve, the heart will just beat like that of a newborn baby.

It takes about six months for the new heart to learn how to respond to the messaging system and eventually slow down a little as well. You must be careful and not allow the new heart to get above 130 bpm's as sometimes it will continue to keep rising and not get the message to slow down again, which has been known to cause a heart attack. For the rest of your life a slow, long warm up and cool down is necessary to keep the heart healthy. My resting heart rate has gone from 120 to 90 bpm's over these past few years.

On the day of moving to the Coronary Care Unit (CCU), I had the ART and PICC lines removed. All I had attached now was a catheter.

Eye of the Tiger
– Survivor

Now on the CCU ward I was allowed more visitors. I felt so lucky to have such a great support network. My friends from work came in, jovial and filling me in on all the gossip of what had been going on at school. Lots of laughs and having fun, feeding me along with helping me drink my cups of tea from a straw. I loved listening to their silly banter and keeping things light. I was never short of having 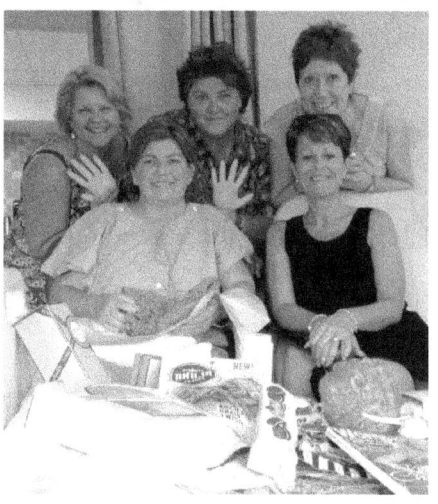 someone come in, usually bringing food they had specially made for me.

I still couldn't eat by myself. I had what they call the 'Tacro shakes'. Tacrolimus is one of the three main anti-rejection drugs and it takes a while for your body to adjust to having it in your system. Your hands shake terribly and trying to hold a cup or spoon to your mouth and get it in is quite a challenge. I remember one day when the occupational therapist (OT) came in to teach me how to clean my teeth. He handed me a glass of water and as I tried to get a mouthful, my teeth were clinking and chattering on the glass. He told me to stop, realising how bad the shakes were but I tried again and with hearing the clinking again, I began laughing. He took the glass from me and as I was joking about it, he laughed too. It was definitely something you had to make light of.

The first few days, the nurses would help me into the chair and I got used to sitting up for a while. I was so weak; I needed a neck support to hold my head up because I got so tired holding it upright for any amount of time. It's amazing how much effort it takes to sit upright in a chair when you've been lying flat for two weeks.

Day four the catheter came out, so I could become more mobile. The first big event of having a real shower was about to take place, very exciting indeed. Being helped into the shower chair, the gorgeous nurse gave me the shower head to hold while she soaped and washed me with a washcloth. She also washed my hair, always a highlight for me. Then she said, 'While I make your bed, why don't you play in the shower like Dumbo?' I could imagine Dumbo the elephant swishing around the water and frolicking in it and that's exactly how I felt with the water running over my body. It was the best feeling ever and most definitely the best shower I have ever had.

I slowly began walking around the ward with a Zimmer frame and the help of the physiotherapist. Short walks along one side of the floor, twice a day was the first stage. Then, when Les or the boys came in, I would get them to come with me for a lap around the ward. I was determined to make good progress. Not being able to see, I knew I would have to learn a lot of new skills, so I was determined to get myself strong enough to make it happen.

Right from when I knew my vision loss was going to be permanent, I focused on getting myself up and running as quickly as possible. I needed to learn how to do basic, everyday tasks by myself, not wanting to be dependent on anyone, especially my family. Just because I had lost my vision, I didn't want life to change for Les or my boys. Their life needed to go on as normal. Mark was in year 11 and Scott had just entered the workforce, they didn't need to be worried about looking after their mother.

When Mum found out about my vision, she contacted Vision Australia. She gave the OT the information about me and she arranged with Mum to come and visit me at the hospital. On her first visit, she taught me the very basics of how to answer my phone using 'voice over'. A simple task like answering a mobile phone soon becomes difficult when you can't see to swipe, to open or answer. Not only was the vision aspect tricky but add in the Tacrolimus tremors and it is nearly impossible.

I'm not going into the nitty gritty of how 'voice over' works but in a nutshell, there are hand gestures to make the phone perform its functions. A one-finger double tap is different to a two-finger double tap and then if you accidently do a three-finger double tap, you make the phone go black. I can tell you now, that for the first few weeks—more like months—I was very frustrated because having the shakes, you don't always make the correct number of taps or fingers for that matter. I also didn't have the knowledge to remember or know how to rectify what I had done to the phone. I was constantly voicing a message to the OT asking how to get my phone functioning with a screen again. The old saying, 'you only learn from your mistakes,' is certainly true. I made a lot of mistakes but learned quickly how to use the phone.

The lovely Vision Australia OT would phone me through the week to see how I was going and came out each week to teach me something else. Along with the taps, there is the same amount of gestures with swipes to do other functions. At least I had the ability to answer my phone to talk to people if they rang. The ball was starting to roll in getting Vision Australia to set me up with IT and in-home function support when I got home.

One of the things that was playing on my mind was the question of, would I be able to return to work in the school? How would I be able to do my job as an Education Assistant when most of the job entails reading and scribing for the children? Then, when two of my friends from school came in to visit, they had the most wonderful news. They told me a discussion was had with the Principal about what had happened to me and my vision. He told them he never had any doubt I wouldn't return to work, even if he had to make a suitable position available for me. He definitely wanted me back, unless I didn't want to return, of course. That was the best news I ever had. It lifted me up so much knowing I would be able to go back to where I loved working, with all my friends and the children.

It was in the fourth week that I was taken to eye clinic at Royal Perth Hospital to get the official testing and report on my sight done. A 'field vision' test, a scan and special types of photos were taken of my eyes. Then, when I saw the Ophthalmologist, he told me I had Ischaemic Optic Neuropathy. Ischaemic means blood vessel, Optic is obviously of the eye and Neuropathy is of the nerve. The blood supply to the Optic Nerve had been damaged through lack of oxygen. Nerves are one of the body tissues that can't be repaired. He said he usually saw it in patients who had initially lost a lot of blood from a sudden trauma. The blood loss is sudden and large but is stopped quickly and usually affects one eye or the other. Also, the vision loss is either top or bottom of your field of vision.

My loss of blood was large but continued over a four-day period. Both my eyes had been affected, both top and bottom. I had about 5% of my right peripheral vision and nothing at all usable in my left. He went on to explain my eyes were still able to function perfectly but the nerve that goes to the part of the brain which tells you how to see things was damaged. The one thing I am truly grateful for is I can still see light, bright colours and large objects. I may not have any clear, defined vision but I'm not in total darkness. That would be another ball game completely and I don't know whether I could have dealt with that so easily. I really have a great deal of respect for those who are totally blind.

Scott had his 18th birthday in the hospital's food hall. Mum made the food at home and bought it in. My brother Geoff, who was still up on the ward, came down to celebrate Scott's birthday. His son Ashley came in too and Eddie, Hon, Les and Mark were all there. I went down in a wheelchair and made the best out of the situation we were in. It turned out to be really nice. Scott unwrapped his gifts and we all enjoyed the hot food Mum had prepared. None of the normal party food was missing. Then a birthday cake appeared and candles were lit and much to Scott's embarrassment, 'Happy Birthday' was sung. At least we were all there as a family to celebrate with him.

I continued to make steady progress and could now walk around the ward floor unsupported. By the end of the second week on the CCU, I was ready for the next lower level of care. I wasn't ready to go home yet and the team knew that, with the vision issue, I would need more support. The rehab centre in the hospital was going to be the best place to continue my recovery.

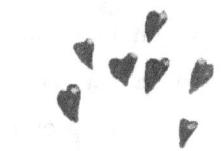

Break My Stride
– Matthew Wilder

At the rehab centre, I soon began a more rigorous exercise program. I was now showering by myself and could eat most meals if the nurse cut up the meat and vegies. I would have to ask what it was on the plate that I was going to eat but at least I was becoming more independent.

Another aspect of life I needed to master was looking after my diabetes. When I was in CCU, the diabetic educator taught me how to dial up the insulin by listening to the clicks. Most of the time the nurses would always check after I had dialled it up to make sure it was the correct dose before injecting it. That part was easy, I had been doing it for 43 years.

When I got to the rehab centre, the diabetic clinic had ordered a talking blood glucose machine for me. It was the same as the other blood glucose monitors I had but this one talked, telling me when it's ready and when to insert the strip. Then when you put the drop of blood on it (which is quite tricky), it reads out the result. At least I could again have independence with my diabetes.

At the rehab gym, the physio set some very basic exercises to do, including some strength and core exercises, along with small bouts of cardio on a bike. The whole time still having my heart rate monitored and blood pressure taken. It felt good to be back doing some exercise, it's always been such a core part of my life.

In addition to the gym, I did some basic exercises in my room each day by myself, trying to gain as much strength as possible. I had to focus on doing things I could do for myself, not only physically but mentally, to keep me staying positive. I still had visitors every day, which was great as it broke up the isolation I was feeling. My brother brought in some audio books with his device, so I could listen to some stories but trying to operate the device was too hard and I would have to get the nurse to turn it on, then switch it off.

By the fourth day of going to the gym, I was pushing myself harder to try and make new gains in my progress. The physio was still supervising me, so I felt confident I was doing well. I was feeling quite proud of myself. After one particular gym session, I began to feel quite unwell at dinner. At that time, Les phoned to ask if I wanted him and Mark to come in for a visit. I told him not to worry as I wasn't feeling very well and wasn't up to making conversation. He told me he would come in and leave Mark at home. He wanted to be with me if I wasn't feeling well.

I told the nurse I couldn't eat anything and needed to lie down. She helped me to bed and asked how I was feeling. I told her I felt strange and weird. Then, as I lay there in bed my legs began to jump and twitch. The nurse watched not knowing what was going on. The leg movements became more violent. This went on for about 15 minutes then the convulsions moved up into my torso. I felt like I had been possessed by a demon. My body was thrashing about in upward, jolting movements.

It was then that Les walked in to see me jumping around in bed. He was shocked and concerned seeing me like that. The nurse was great, keeping me reassured, even though she had no idea what was happening. She called the doctor. She saw I was sweating and got a nice cold flannel and kept wiping my face and the back of my neck. I began to get really tired, my muscles were having a hard training session all by themselves.

Les tried holding my legs down to see if that helped but as those muscles were restrained, my upper body increased its movement. My back was lifting off the mattress and it was more uncomfortable. Then he held my body down and my legs began to thrash harder. It was a no-win situation.

I remember the intense fatigue I was feeling but had no control to stop my muscles from moving. It had been going on for over an hour and I had no idea how long it would continue.

The doctor came in and after asking some questions, took some blood while the nurse held my arm still. He was completely baffled as to what was going on. He couldn't give me anything because he didn't know what was causing it and any additional medication may interfere with the transplant drugs.

It was now about 10 pm, and after a three-hour uncontrollable exercise session, my body finally decided to give in. Stillness resumed and a huge sigh of relief had by all of us. Completely exhausted, I just wanted to go to sleep. Les finally went home and watching him leave, I was so glad he did come in. It would have been very unnerving going through that by myself.

Every few hours through the night, my body would start up again and I would call the nurse. She just told me to breathe and try and relax. It only lasted for a few minutes and then subsided. I just didn't want it to happen again.

In the morning when the transplant team came around, they did some tests on my muscle movement. My legs were still twitching a little. They got me up to go for a walk. My balance was a bit shaky, so Dr A held my hand for a bit. Then the weirdest thing happened. When I took my first step, it was an over exaggerated movement. I couldn't control it, though. The muscles seemed to have a mind of their own, raising the leg up high before coming down. The doctors were dumbfounded by what they were seeing. I felt like a prancing pony. The only explanation they could come up with was the extra intensity in the gym the day before was too much for my muscles to deal with. With everything that had gone on over the last month, my muscles would have to slowly regain their memory as well. They told me to just take it slow and not to overdo it in the gym.

Mark came in with Les that night to be reassured I was OK. I showed him what happened when I put my feet on the floor. Sitting on my bed, as my toes touched the floor they began to tap. My feet performed an uncontrolled tap-dancing sequence by merrily tapping up and down all by themselves. I imagined myself as Ginger Rogers wearing a glittery silver dress that dazzled under the shining lights (perhaps not with the red hair, though), tap dancing up on a glamorous stage with Fred Astaire. We were all cracking up laughing. You really couldn't do anything but have fun with it. Mark recorded it on his phone and sent it to a girlfriend, saying, 'Look at Mum's tap-dancing feet.'

Les took me for a walk that night and the best way I can describe my gait was that I was prancing like some sort of awkward, gawky, gazelle or doing a John Cleese 'Ministry of Funny Walks' impersonation with my high-lifting strides. I was embarrassed, to be honest but Les assured me it was nothing to be embarrassed about. True love.

The following day, my muscles decided to behave themselves again. I was once again back in the gym at an easier pace, rebuilding my muscle strength and gaining the bit I had lost over the past two days.

During the whole stay in hospital, Eddie would visit every day, put me in the wheelchair and push me all around the outside of the hospital and through the garden paths, describing what things looked like and what we were passing. Stephen managed to be brought over each week for a visit and he also pushed me around the garden areas while we chatted about his progress and what he was doing in rehab. Mum was there every day in the morning when everyone else was at work. Hon visited every other day after work. She was by my side through this whole ordeal. I have always loved her bright and happy disposition, we had good laughs; growing up together, we always had a strong connection. My brother David came in when he was down from his FIFO work. I knew he had been there when I was in the ICU as he also entered my nightmare.

Les and Mark would usually come after school or when Les got home from his job. Scott drove in after work to see me, which was nice as we had our own time together. If they were there at the same time, both Scott and Mark would fight over who was going to push me in the wheelchair when we went down to the food hall for a drink. It was lovely to be fought over in such a loving way. I was always surrounded by so many people who loved me so much, truly a blessing indeed.

One day, Mum bought Jasper, our little pet dog, down. While she waited at the coffee shop outside of the hospital building, Les and the boys came and wheeled me down. I had no idea they had brought Jasper in. When we got to the coffee shop, Mum handed me Jasper and put him on my lap. He had been so stressed not understanding why I was not at home with Les and the boys and so upset during the previous few weeks. It was so lovely holding him again. It must be incredibly hard on pets when they have no way of knowing what has happened or why a person is missing from the family. I truly think Jasper aged a lot over the six weeks I was in hospital.

Plans were now being put in place for my return home. Both Vision Australia and the hospital were liaising on how to move forward. The social worker had also been doing a lot of support work enquiries and getting them signed and approved before I left the hospital.

Six weeks to the day, I went home.

Welcome Back
– John Sebastian

Finally, home again with my family. At first, settling in at home was a little stressful. Les was on the boys telling them to keep things out of walkways so I wouldn't trip over. Everyone was on tenterhooks worrying how things would go and what things I could do for myself. I wanted to go into our pool for a swim as it was still very hot in the middle of February. Les helped me into the pool area and held my hand for balance as I walked down the steps into the water. He told Mark to stay outside and watch me in case I drowned. I told him I may not be able to see but I could still swim. That was how worried and paranoid Les was about something happening to me. I guess he just didn't want to entertain the thought of losing me after it had already come so close before. I felt the stress he was holding within himself, poor love.

Les also had the new career label of 'Pharmacist'. The hospital had done up a coloured chart of all my medications and when to take them. Initially, I was on 25 tablets morning and night. Plus, I had to be weighed every day to check I wasn't gaining any fluid. If that happened, I had to ring the hospital and tell them and take a diuretic. This was really important as it could be a sign the heart is not working properly. After a week or so, things slowly settled down as a new routine began.

Les had become efficient with cooking with the boys at night. My girlfriends would also bring around meals to help Les with the cooking side of things. He would make my toast and cup of tea for breakfast and get the house all sorted for the day. I was still weak and unable to eat much at all for quite a few months. The boys seemed happier I was home again and we were all back as a family unit. Life was starting to return to normal.

Being immunosuppressed, I wasn't allowed out in public for about three months. Infection is easy to catch and hard to cure. My friends would call around and have a cuppa and a catch-up, which was always welcome. Once Les had returned to work, Mum would come each day to get my lunch and help with anything that needed doing. Most of the day I would listen to the radio. I began practicing walking up and down our driveway then around the house. After a week or so, I thought I would attempt our outside stairs. That was a bit tricky. I held onto the limestone wall, as balance was quite an issue. I counted six steps, then a landing before the next six steps to the bottom. Coming up is always easier than going down, even now. When I told Les I went down the stairs that day, he was very impressed. He knew I was trying to do everything I could to improve.

It was Monday of the third week and Clare phoned me to see how I was doing. I told her for the past four days I had been really tired. Even after breakfast, I needed to lie down on the couch and sleep. She knew that wasn't normal for me at all. She told me to come in right away so they could check me out and see what was going on. Mum drove me to the hospital and once they saw me, they admitted me. After running some bloods, it became clear my blood cells were all beginning to mutate. The tiredness was caused by my low oxygen levels, with fewer red blood cells to transport it round my system. It turns out it was caused by one of the drugs I was on. Long story short, two blood transfusions later and I began to pick up again, albeit slowly. I was home again one week later.

I continued improving and doing tasks by myself. Things started to pick up. A strange thing had been happening since I returned home and I guess it is common after what I'd been through. I would have dreams of my vision returning and would wake up with tears in my eyes once I realised it was only a dream. The dreams ranged from happy experiences to ones of having to tell everyone I could see again and I had been a fraud all this time, just trying to gain attention. It was quite unnerving when I had them but with time, they were less frequent.

I'm thinking it just must take some time for your brain to re-adjust to suddenly not having a sense to help navigate the surrounding environment. Most probably, your subconsciousness must have to catch up with what your conscious mind is now dealing with in a new reality. I don't know but that's my take on it.

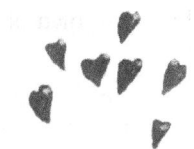

Tubthumping
- Chumbawamba

It was the Easter long weekend and we had nice things planned. On the Good Friday night, I had a bit of a temperature but when I woke in the morning I felt fine. The day was uneventful, then that night I again had a temperature with a few shivers and shakes but when I got up in the morning, I felt OK again. We enjoyed Easter Sunday with Amanda and Paul along with Mum, Scott and Mark, who drove us to an Easter country fair. Our friends told me that I didn't look well. I said, of course, I was fine. Sunday night and I wasn't feeling quite right and again through the night ran another fever. Monday morning, I sat trying to make idle conversation but knew I had to go to the hospital. I felt bad as Stephen was to come out for the day and he wanted to share it with me and the family, even though he said he completely understood. He still had the boys to talk to and do things with at home.

Les took me to the hospital and after being admitted and having bloods run, I got quite a lecture from the team as to why didn't I come in on the Saturday after the first bout of having a temperature. I said I felt fine through the day but didn't want to spoil the Easter weekend by landing in hospital again. The initial results came back as a kidney infection, so I began a course of antibiotics. However, further testing showed it was an E. coli infection that had got into my blood stream. That was not good, so along with another lecture of how it could have been prevented with early admittance, I was on a course of intravenous antibiotics. I spent another week in hospital.

You are informed before the transplant that the first six months are a wipe off, having the first six biopsies weekly, followed by three a fortnight apart, then once a month for three months. Not only the biopsies but any drugs that don't suit you, or contracting an infection always results in another hospital stay. I guess in the big scheme of it all, you have been given a second precious chance at life and that is certainly a good reason for a little inconvenience in the first six or so months.

During this time, Vision Australia had been coming and organising special things that would make my life easier. I ordered a long cane and had a practice with one to know how to use it and what it felt like. When it came time to choosing a cane, I asked if they came in any other colour but white. They told me black was also an option. I told them I don't do black. I didn't want to have a typical white blind cane. If I'm having one, I'm doing it in style.

The OT's thought this was funny and after doing a bit of research in their catalogues, they found a fluoro yellow and a hot pink cane with a purple ball on the tip. Oh yeah, baby. I'll work that little number just fine. Excitedly, they ordered the hot pink cane for me.

I didn't want to be defined by my blindness. I wasn't going to just go along with the stereotypical image of a blind person. I was going to be proud and make a statement of it. I always dressed in nice bright coloured clothes and wore the latest fashions with the help of my dear girlfriend's, Jane and Dee, alias Trinny and Susannah. We had a lot of fun shopping. They would scout around the clothes store and choose a few items each, take me into the change room and help me try on the clothes. Since the transplant, it was necessary to buy a new wardrobe because I had dropped over ten kilograms, so unbelievably, I was now a size eight. I felt great and ready to step out in my new wardrobe.

I had in-home support now in the form of a lovely carer who helped me organise my pantry, laundry and bathroom cupboards so I could find items I needed and know the difference between containers of similar shape and size.

She would also take me for a walk around the local streets and around our nearby park. I hadn't been able to walk to this park for over a year now as my old heart couldn't make the distance. Now I was able to walk up there and all around the paths, then back home again. It did feel good indeed.

Having a lot of time at home by myself, I soon began to fill it with exercise. I had always done resistance training as part of my lifestyle routine, so I began building my fitness up again. Les showed me how to put on a CD that I could exercise to. Then I was off and running, doing my weight training. I started off easy, then obtained a few more coloured weights I could see, to make things easier. Eventually, I would do an hour's resistance training each day, which felt amazing. I could feel myself gaining muscle definition and strength once more, good old muscle memory had come to my rescue.

I needed to add in cardio to compliment my workout. Having walked twice up to the park now with my support worker, I wasn't going to wait for her once a week to get some walking in. I felt confident enough to venture out by myself. For the first two outings, I never told Les or Mum I was going on a walk by myself. I knew they would be beside themselves worrying about what could happen to me. What they didn't know wouldn't hurt them, was my thinking.

I initially took Jasper and just walked up to the park and then would do multiple laps within that space. It soon became a bit boring and I needed a bit more of a challenge with some hills in it. Very easy to get a hill workout living up in Lesmurdie, in the Darling Ranges of Perth. I was soon walking five kilometres a day and quickly extended out to eight kilometres, with hills.

My fitness was really escalating quickly and I was feeling like Wonder Woman. Perhaps imagine that without the red shorts and vibrant blue top and take away the gold headband too but that was what I felt like and I was loving it.

When people found out I was walking by myself, they were quite shocked, asking if I got scared or worried? My reply was, 'You only hit things once and you soon remember where they are and don't hit them again.' I had quite a few good bruises on my left arm. Bus stops, bollards and signposts were always wanting to jump out and say hello to me but I only engaged in the conversation with them once or twice. I also had no depth perception, so falling or tripping down curbs or uneven ground was challenging too.

With all the walking and navigating my environment, I began having neck and shoulder issues from constantly having to turn my head to the left and down to try and make things out to the side of where I was going. But nothing was going to hold me back. I was a steam train powering forward.

It was now May, and my dear friend Katharine from school asked if I would like to try yoga. It could be something to participate in a group and something different to try. None of us had done yoga before so it would be new to all of us. Jane from work was also coming along. Katharine checked with the instructor first to ask if it was alright for me to come and she was more than happy for me to come and try.

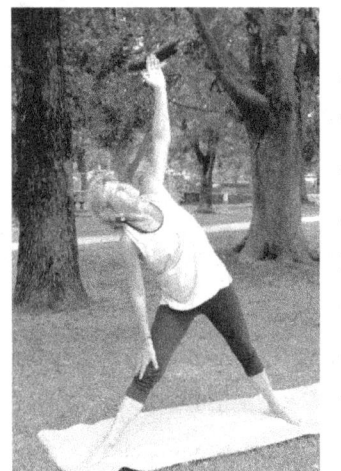

To cut a long story short, Katharine still picks me up and takes me to yoga to this day. We had lots of laughs and giggles during the first few months with the challenging positions, particularly the moves containing a balancing component. Not so long ago, Katharine told me she and Jane were worried about me, not so much my sight but my heart dropping out onto the floor while doing the downward dog. A joke they privately shared.

I never did anything but make fun of the things that went on in the secure zone of that sacred Zen space. Katharine and Jane also made fun of me, which lightened things up for everyone there. Tammy, the yoga instructor, always said she loved my energy and having me in the class. I'm not sure about the other participants, though.

Tammy is a compassionate, gentle soul. I always leave her class feeling totally calm and rejuvenated.

Katharine was one of those friends I had a special connection with. I could easily open up to her and knew she understood. It's funny how you can have a range of very special friends you connect with at certain levels but then you get the one or two that somehow have a deeper connection and understanding. Some you don't say things to as they get worried too easily, while others listen but you feel it's been lost in translation. However, their love and support are unwavering.

I remember Katharine picking me up one day to take me to have coffee with the girls and she asked me how I was doing, *really*? Really, I felt like a fraud. She asked me what I meant. I told her I thought to be blind it had to be a total black out; I could still see light, shapes and colours to some degree. I'm classified as legally blind but I can still see a bit. She laughed and said just because I had about 5% peripheral vision on one side and what I do see is not clear, did I think that didn't count? Sitting there listening to her put it in to perspective how little I could see and do, made me feel a little better. I found out from Vision Australia only 3% of the blind population are totally blind. I felt somewhat better then.

My weight had continued to drop each week until I finally bottomed out at 55 kgs. That was a bit too low but I wasn't doing it deliberately. I was still eating only very small amounts. Then when I did eventually begin to eat a little more, I was exercising morning, noon and night. It was the only thing I had to focus on and now I had yoga stretches to add into my routine throughout the day. I loved working out, I always felt so good afterwards.

A couple of months after being home from the transplant, Dad came to visit. He was so pleased to see me up and about doing all the things I did before, like hanging out washing and making him a cup of coffee. I guess he must have thought he would find me sitting in my chair waiting for someone to make me a cup of tea and do everything for me.

After catching up on how I was going, I began to tell him about my nightmare. This was common for me early on to tell friends about parts of it, it was still very fresh and imprinted on my mind. As I unravelled parts of this nonsensical alternate life I lived, I told him I didn't understand it. I am such a positive person, I should have been in Willy Wonka Land with the chocolate river and all the scrumptious lollies, not hell on earth.

He sat there in complete awe of this story and told me how pleased he was I had shared it with him. Not only did he find it intriguing of how the brain still works in an unconscious state but there was not one part of the story where I was either not fighting for my life or my family's life. I was fighting a conspiracy or fighting an injustice of some kind. He told me that was me fighting for my life.

After that, I viewed the nightmare in a completely different light and could now see how I was mentally having an internal battle to stay alive. It took Dad to pick out the purpose of the grim and wretched state I had lived through. No one else, not even me, had seen that.

Thank you, Dad, for bringing light to a dark reality.

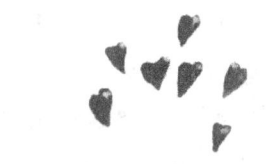

Don't Stop Me Now
– Queen

Big adjustments were experienced by my whole family. I had gone from being slow and sickly prior to the transplant to near death and then blind. Everybody close to me had been on a roller-coaster ride of stress and worry. I felt for them all and appreciate the loving support they gave me throughout the weeks and months of all that uncertainty.

Now, as I recovered, I became a headstrong, wild woman who was taking on everything she could find. I was wanting to go out dancing, listen to music and make the most out of life. It was as if the Grim Reaper had missed his chance of getting me for the second time and I was not going to let anything stand in my way of making the most of it. I felt invincible and to sit on the lounge at night watching TV was too much of a waste of precious time.

Unbeknown to me, this new-found energy and verve for life was taking its toll on Les. One day, I walked into the office and found him sitting with his head in his hands, leaning on the table. He didn't move when I entered. I asked, what was the matter? Distressed and teary, he said he couldn't keep up with me. He said how I was wanting to do so many things, exercising, yoga, kayaking and riding around the river on a tandem, wanting to go out all the time and he was too tired to go out and do all these things with me. He worked long hours and had been keeping the house going and I was now this unstoppable energetic person wanting to make the most out of life. He totally understood why I would be feeling that way, especially with losing my vision and not being able to get out by myself but he just couldn't keep up.

I hadn't stopped to think how my behaviour had been affecting him. I felt terrible. I told him I didn't expect for him to have to keep up. I just wanted to go out with the girls and have fun with them, as long as he didn't mind. That really strengthened our relationship. I realised how much stress he had been dealing with, which I had never even thought about. I had been so self-consumed with charging ahead with life, Les felt as if I was leaving him behind. Even the boys were trying to keep up with my comings and goings, it must have been difficult for them to deal with as well.

I don't know if it is the same with all transplant patients but you feel you have been given this second chance of life and not a minute of it is going to be wasted. Time is too precious and there is so much to experience to enjoy out there, you just want to make the most of it. This new-found energy just keeps rising in you and the only option I found was to charge along with it.

I was always thinking of what else I could do. Typical aerobics were out as I couldn't see what the instructor was doing. Then I thought about swimming. I had enough vision to be able to follow the black line on the bottom of the pool. I hadn't swum for 20 years, what with frozen shoulders and surgery and not being able to get my arms up over my head, swimming had not been on my exercise radar.

But God works in mysterious ways indeed. Whether it was because I had my chest cracked open for four days and/or being in a coma that all my muscles and tendons were relaxed and able to stretch, I don't know. While I was in the CCU an amazing thing happened. I was sitting on my bed and just happened to stretch my arms up over my head. Suddenly, realising what I had just done, I began to move my arms in full rotation to see what they could do. I was so excited; you have no idea. Not only did I have a new heart but I had a body that was now fully functional. Perhaps the universe thought, if we're giving her a new engine, we had better rebuild the chassis as well. I was now a hot V8 race car and painted red because we all know red cars go faster.

Then I thought I'd try another impossible task I hadn't been able to do for the past two years. I crossed my legs over. It sounds ridiculous but I had always exercised but never stretched much and then in the last two years, begun sitting more due to health issues, so my hip flexors tightened up so much I couldn't even cross my legs without immense pain. Now I could do that as well. Going through this whole ordeal was just about worth it to be able to have my flexibility back and improved.

It was after the July school holidays when I asked Les to take me down to the heated pool in Bayswater. I had bought some bathers and goggles prior to getting myself prepared for my next exciting venture. The first time, he came into the pool with me. I got myself ready, feeling a little nervous at first as to how my shoulders would go and just how much I would be able to see.

At first, I just bobbed down to get a bearing of how things would be under water. I stuck my head up and then put it under again.

'Well that's weird. I can see better under water. What the hell's going on?' I said to Les.

'Are you sure? What do you mean you can see better?' he asked.

'The line is clear and defined but when I stick my head up out of the water, it's back to normal vision with not being able to see anything again.' I was now feeling more confident because I could see the black line, though the distance of vision was still very limited to maybe one metre ahead of my view.

I began my first lap. It felt great being in the water. It was as if I had found my new safe and happy place to be. I did a few laps of freestyle and some breaststroke. Les was happy for me, knowing there was something else I was able to do to get out of the house and enjoy.

It didn't take me long at all before I had a routine with Mum taking me to the pool on a regular basis. She would line me up to the lane and tell me if it was free or how many people were in it. While I did my laps, she went over to the smaller pool and walked in the walking lanes to get her exercise in as well.

I quickly built up to swimming 1600 metres. Switching it up with flippers, a buoy for my legs to build up my arms and introducing backstroke to my repertoire as well. I was in seventh heaven. Swimming three days a week, weight training alternate days and walking every day. My energy levels were going through the roof. I was really feeling back in the game now.

Just six months after my operation, sometime around June, I thought I would try to start doing some cooking. Using a crock pot would be the safest option until my confidence in the kitchen improved. I could at least make my toast putting butter and jam on it, making quite a mess, mind you but at least I was doing it for myself. Sometimes Mark would say, 'Mum, stop. Let me do it. You're getting it everywhere but on the toast.' I would let him do it as it would stress him out seeing the sticky mess I was making. Pouring a cup of tea could become quite a disaster in no time at all with either the boiling water or the milk not making it into the cup. Today, however, I am quite good at it, only missing the milk occasionally. If you come for a cuppa, you need to be prepared to only get half a cup of coffee as I don't like using the squealy water level gauge I was given. It's too noisy.

Getting back to my cooking attempts, Mum would come and help cut and peel the vegetables with me, get the ingredients I was needing and then watch as I got it all together. After a couple of times, I attempted the whole process myself. I cut the vegies up and yes, they may have been interesting shapes and sizes. I then opened what I thought was tinned tomatoes and trying to empty the contents into the crock pot, nothing came out. So, I put in a teaspoon to get it out and it was solid. I had a sniff, it didn't have a smell I recognised. So, into the tin I delved and took a mouthful and soon spat it out. It was kidney beans. Not something I usually eat cold from the tin. I found another tin in the cupboard and opened it and that one was the tomatoes.

Les got home from work that night and I had the table already set. I told him I had cooked dinner all by myself and it was all ready. He and the boys sat down at the dinner table. They dished up and after a few mouthfuls the critique was very favourable indeed. Making quite a fuss about what a great job I had done. Between you and me, I think they were just glad not to have to do the cooking for a change.

Even today, a few ingredients are substituted accidently. If I can't be bothered using the technology that enables label reading and I just wing it, thinking I know that's what the ingredient feels like, I just put it in. We had a banana cake one weekend made with breadcrumbs instead of almond meal. It didn't turn out too bad either, just a little different in texture. It's not too often the boys won't eat what's on offer.

Even though I'm back to doing most of the cooking again, Les will walk into the kitchen occasionally and say, 'Ahh. You've been cooking again, dear.'

'Yes, I've got dinner all ready and I've made a banana cake,' would be my excited announcement. 'I even cleaned all the kitchen up, too.'

'Very good dear, I can see that. I might just get the bits you've missed,' he'd respond kindly, knowing I've tried my best in doing something I always did so easily. Then he would be there for about ten minutes cleaning the stove top, splash backs and benches. Never ever complaining, he just got in there and finished the job properly. I do love him for always being just so loving and understanding. The boys are great, too. Seeing my mess, they'd say, 'Mum, just leave it. We'll do it,' and never in an angry tone. All the men in my life are very patient and understanding. I'm so grateful to be blessed with such loving people.

Being able to eat my meals by myself was becoming easier. The first few weeks at home, Les and the boys would tell me where things were on the plate. Potato is at 12 o'clock, peas are at 3, meat is at 6, carrots at 9, would be the description. One night, I was trying to stab some carrots onto my fork. Scott was saying, 'Nearly, no, a bit more to the right. Nearly, no more to the top. I've never seen anyone stab all over the plate and hit everywhere but where they're meant to,' he said, quite amused and intrigued with my amazing missing attempts.

'For God's sake, just put the bloody carrots on my fork for me,' I would say, while making fun of the situation.

Scott responded, 'You wouldn't be much good at playing battleships, Mum.' We all made light of the things that happened, it was the only way to be able to stay positive and happy.

I remember asking the Vision OT one day, 'How do you ever eat out in public without making a huge mess cutting up your own food and not getting it all over the table?'

She told me, 'At first, just eat finger food you can pick up. It can be tricky even for those who have been blind for a long time. You do get to know what to order out and what is just too hard.'

Sometimes, when we would go out for dinner with friends, I would feel like a child, having Les cut up my steak or schnitzel but it was the only way I could eat what I felt like having. Sometimes I would get cranky and tell him, 'I can do it.'

He would say, 'Have a go but I can tell you now, the plate is full and there's not much room for error.'

Reluctantly I would give in and let him do it as I would feel worse if I spilled my food all over the table. It wasn't a major dilemma but for someone who was always so very independent, having people cut up your food and help you eat it felt quite deflating at times.

I'm pleased to say I can now eat almost anything with confidence out in public. I don't mind using my fingers, if needed, sometimes it's the only way to safely get meat away from the bones. Occasionally, someone might suggest I cut what's on my fork as it might not fit in my mouth but I feel quite confident that if I were to be 'fine dined' I would pass the proper social etiquette standards.

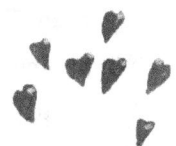

Walking on Sunshine
- Katrina and the Waves

Several months after my transplant, I went with Mum to a 'Write to your donor family day' hosted by Donate Life. These events are an opportunity to meet other recipients and to get guidance on writing to your donor family, as the recipient of their loved one's organ. As you would expect, there are privacy and confidentiality issues, as well as things that are appropriate and not appropriate to include in the correspondence. We were guided through the process to help us put down in our own words, our thoughts and our gratitude. By all accounts, these letters are generally well received by the families of the organ donor. I suppose it's living and written proof their loved one's loss of life has given life to another. Another who is sincerely grateful. Another who's family and loved one's are also sincerely grateful and humbled by such an awesome gift.

As with everything that was happening to me, it was great meeting others who had been through similar journeys to myself and hear their stories. Many of those in our group had suffered and were still suffering from guilt and depression. This is a common reaction to having an organ transplant. I felt for these people. Yes, I had experienced days of depression, of finding it difficult to see any light at the end of the tunnel but I did what I've done with all the challenges life has thrown at me—picked myself up, looked the challenge in the eye, and said, 'You are not going to beat me.' So, while I did have some depression, my own reaction was one of overwhelming gratitude coupled with renewed energy and verve for life that even I was finding challenging to exhaust.

It was during this meeting at the 'Write to your donor family day' that I found out about the 'Transplant Games', a sporting competition exclusively for people who have had an organ transplant. The Australian games are held every second year and the World games every other year. The next games were in 2018 on the Gold Coast in Queensland. Instantly, on hearing of these games, I knew what my destiny was to be. It was a light bulb moment and I immediately commenced planning in my head what I needed to do to compete in the swimming events, realising too, it would be another awesome goal for me to achieve and a brilliant physical challenge to keep me motivated and focused while I was still recovering and waiting to get back to work.

When I told a few friends, they all jumped on the band wagon with me. Super supportive and excited. My dear friend Tracy, who was also my Bowen therapist since before the transplant, set up a 'Go Fund Me' fundraiser principally because I would have to take someone with me if Les couldn't get time off work. The daunting thought of navigating the airport, plane and then getting around was a bit out of my realm.

It was not long after I had decided to take on the games that there was a notice through Transplant Australia asking if anyone would like to apply for the TV show 'This time next year'. They must have had a recent transplant and have a goal they were trying to achieve.

Straight away, I replied and after a few phone calls and conversations of my story so far, I was put on the list to be confirmed later by the TV show. I never said anything to anyone just in case it didn't happen.

From this contact with Transplant Australia, my story was forwarded to 'That's Life' magazine as they were requesting a transplant story for their 'Donate Life' week campaign. I was contacted by the magazine and after sending them some photos, I was the promotional awareness story. Vision Australia was also looking for some interviews to put in their newsletter, so guess who was photographed with her bright hot-pink cane? By the way, I was the first person in Western Australia to have a coloured cane like that. Even the OTs were excited and impressed when they opened the box containing this trendy, amazing cane, soon to be desired and admired by the blind community.

It was Mark's 17th birthday, and I was getting all the party food organised for dinner. Clare called me with the results from the bloods I had done the day before. She told me my kidneys were through the roof and my Tacro level was extremely high. What had I taken different in the previous few days? All I could think of was an over-the-counter drug I'd purchased because I had some thrush.

'Oh No! you can't take anything like that without checking with the pharmacist first. Did they ask you if you had any medical history?'

'No.'

'You may not like what I'm going to say but we think you need to come into hospital. We need to flush the Tacro out of your system with diuretics and watch how your kidneys go.'

'It's Mark's birthday and I've got all the food ready. Can I come in the morning, surely one night won't make any difference?'

'I'll check with Dr A but I don't like your chances,' she replied.

About two hours later, Dr A phoned and said, 'We've got a bed ready for you. How long until you can get here?'

'Can I come in the morning?'

'No. When Tacro levels go really high like that and the drug that caused it is still in your system, it can continue to climb. Your kidneys don't like Tacro at the best of times and quite quickly, you could go into kidney failure. We don't won't that to happen,' he told me. 'We need to start treating you tonight to start getting the Tacro level down. Sorry, but you know how these things go.'

I packed my bag, told Mark when Dad got home I had to go into hospital but Nanna would still come down for his birthday dinner. It was only fair since Scott had to have his 18th in hospital. Karma certainly has her way with keeping the status quo. She never ceases to amaze me how she keeps things balanced.

I spent five days in hospital while they introduced a new drug that would complement the Tacrolymus and they could lower the amount of Tacro in my system to help my kidneys. This drug was also one they commonly used when another anomaly occurs within the blood vessels of the heart in transplant patients. It would already be in my system to hopefully prevent it from happening as well.

It was about three months later when I had some routine bloods done and my white cell count was extremely low. Being brought back into clinic for review and running more bloods, they discovered the new drug was causing a disruption in my bone marrow function enabling white cell production. Now I was referred on to haematology for further investigation and to be able to get the injections needed to get my white cell production up and running again. Some of my other drugs were reduced as I now had no immune system at all and had to be careful going out in public again. It took a few months to get my white cell count back to normal. Then it was the slow introduction of the main antirejection drugs, because when I started taking them, the cell count would drop once more. Eventually, we got back to normal. It is certainly a fine balancing act to keep things on an even keel as possible.

While all this was happening, I was continuing with my regime of medications and having regular blood tests. I'm not trying to trivialise these events but suffice to say, when you have a transplant of such significant proportions and you are a type 1 diabetic, getting the balance of medications exactly right is a challenge.

At one of my hospital check-ups, Dr A seemed quite upset seeing me and said, 'It's a shame about what happened. Even now, when we bring you up at the meeting each week, we all question if it the right thing to do...'

'Dr A, no regrets. I don't ever regret for one moment what happened. I'm alive, back doing the things I love. Swimming, learning things in a new way. Don't ever think I regret what happened. I'm incredibly grateful for being given the transplant.'

'Only you would have been able to pull off what happened. Even for getting through it alive, let alone how you've dealt with losing your sight. I don't think anyone else would be coping as well as you. You always have been very positive and just get on with things,' he answered.

In September of the year after my transplant, it was coming up to Les and my 20th wedding anniversary. I wanted to give Les a real surprise. After all the stress he had gone through with me, adjustments he had made to his life, all without a murmur of complaint, so it would be nice to arrange something special. Earlier on in the year, I had tried pop quizzing him on, 'If he could have a holiday somewhere, where would he go?' Every place I suggested, like Sydney, Melbourne, the Gold Coast and Tasmania, he said, 'No.' So I had to make the executive decision and with the help of Hon, the Gold Coast was the winner. I secretly asked his boss about getting the time off and requested he keep a 'cone of silence' on the matter and not say anything to him. Then through Frequent Flyer points, I managed to get the flights and hotel all for nothing. Excellent. Everything was booked and between us, Hon and I had concocted a plan of having Les take her to the airport.

Right up to the week before we were to depart, Les had no idea. Then the remarks from the blokes at work got him curious and baffled as to why they were asking where was he going on holiday? Having to get another driver to replace him, word soon got around that he wouldn't be there for a week. So, as you can imagine, the 'cat was out of the bag' and I had to reveal what I had organised and how it was going to play out. He was pretty impressed when I had an answer to all the questions he asked. He tried to fight it but after a few days, once he had time to adjust to the idea, he became like a little kid excited about going on a holiday.

We had an absolutely wonderful time together. Discovering all the wonderful things to do, see and dine out together. We explored the new G-link, a light tram service that was being installed for the Commonwealth games the following year. It was so nice reconnecting with each other after everything that had gone on in the past 12 months. Les had to admit he really enjoyed the time away together and a break from life. It was a much-needed break for both of us.

It was now October and life was going ahead in leaps and bounds. I had increased my training regime in the water, as well as weight training to gain further strength. During this time, Vision Australia sent out our local Seeing Eye

Dog instructor to do an assessment on me, which is a requirement before applying for an assistance animal. As you would expect, there are rigorous guidelines and suitability requirements that must be met. After quite a long interview and assessment, I was told I would be a great candidate for having a Seeing Eye Dog, or SED as we call them for short. I was excited and apprehensive at the same time, not knowing if I would use the dog much and how much hassle it would be having one.

The information was sent to Melbourne to the Seeing Eye Dog headquarters and where the dog training takes place. I was told there were about 50 people already on the list and it may take up to a year before one became available. I was still moving forward.

A few weeks later, the TV show contacted me to hear my story. After going through everything to date, even being on the wait list for a dog, they thought it would be a beautiful and uplifting story to tell. I was super excited but was also told I had to keep it secret. Except for Les, Scott, Mark and Hon, no one else knew. There were pages and pages of contractual agreements to sign. Then it was all official, I was going on the show. Talk about rolling on down the tracks of life full steam ahead. I don't think you can get much fuller than that.

The show got back to me a few weeks later and told me I had to make a pledge. What? A pledge? Not understanding, they explained people came on the show pledging to achieve something in the coming year and the story is followed and filmed throughout the next 12 months. At the end of the 12 months, you return to announce whether or not you have honoured your pledge. It doesn't matter if you don't succeed, it's the story of trying that is the focus. It had to be quite specific, so after a bit of brainstorming my pledge was, 'This time next year, I will win gold at the Transplant Games.' Talk about pressure. Not just competing in them but now I had to win GOLD. Bring it on.

Christmas came and was celebrated with a feeling of gratitude that I was still here and doing extremely well. Our Christmas is always poolside, Hon and her mum and sister always share Christmas with us. We all share in the food preparation and after lunch, you will find us in the pool for the rest of the afternoon, with music, food and laughter, just enjoying each other's company. Les and the boys usually join us in the pool for a while and sometimes even Mum will decide to try out the water but Hon is a real water baby and never wants to get out. A true Zen 'master of water wallowing' is Hon.

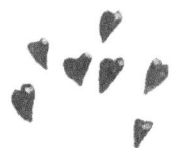

Don't Stop Believin'
– Journey

January 2018, and it was time for my one-year anniversary check up at the hospital. I got to see Dr A, which was so lovely. I always have a deep sense of gratitude to him for seeing the potential in me for a transplant, beyond the statistics that made me a poor medical risk. He had fought bringing my case to the table week after week, when his colleagues believed the risk of conducting a transplant on a type 1 diabetic was a risk they were not willing to take. For the first six months of my clinic meetings, it was always just Dr A and me. It felt like a battle we were fighting by ourselves. You soon feel a real connection when you feel like someone is there when the stakes you're playing are for your life.

He was pleased to see and hear how well I was going. I filled him in on all the things I had been up to. He is always impressed how positive, bubbly and excited I am about life and the challenges I'm

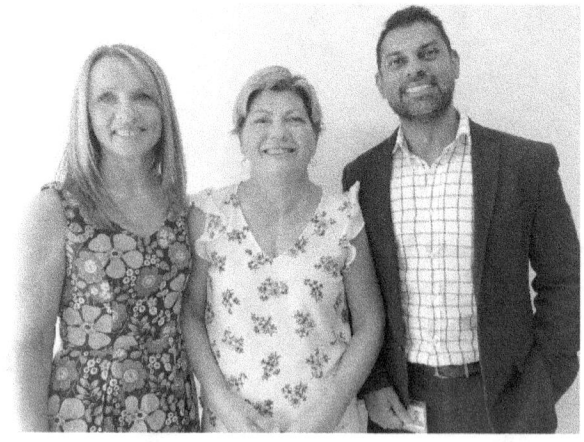

attempting. He did try and tell me to slow down a little but knew that wasn't going to happen, so he just told me to keep doing whatever it was I was doing. He had a huge smile on his face the whole time, which made me feel great. I guess I never wanted him to feel bad about what had happened.

Throughout the year, I would send little videos to Clare showing some of the things I had been getting up to. One was when I had an outing with Vision Australia to the 'I fly' experience, where you can simulate parachuting and fly as though you've jumped out of a plane. It was a great feeling, flying and floating by yourself. Jumping out of a plane is still something I want to do and on my 'to do' list. Another time, Dee had taken me into the Perth food night markets. It was buzzing with people, food and music. Hearing the Latin rhythm in the distance, I said to Dee, 'Let's go and have a listen.' Standing there, listening to the mesmerizing Latin music was just too much. I folded up my pink cane, handed it to Dee and began dancing. I was euphoric. These were the sorts of videos I would send Clare to show the team, usually with the caption 'No regrets'.

On my actual anniversary day, we decided to have a 1st birthday party. All my friends came and we set it up as any princess would celebrate her 1st birthday. It's when I saw everyone together that I became overwhelmed with how much love and support I had. I'm truly and deeply grateful for that, always. I wouldn't have got through the year without all their support and them keeping my spirits up.

Everyone has played some sort of role with helping me, between keeping me in suitable trendy fashion, doing my hair with colour and highlights, not forgetting the especially important task of keeping my eyebrows tamed so I didn't have a caterpillar living on my forehead. Taking me out for lunches and rides around the river on a tandem bike, then venturing into a tandem kayak (thanks to Dee, aka Sporty Spice). These were all things that kept me going, kept me upbeat and looking towards the future in that first year. Even today, as I write this, my wonderful friends are all still keeping me included, looking the part and sharing good times together. I love them all for their unique and quirky ways of showing how they love and value me as a friend. I only hope they feel the love, gratitude and respect I have for them in return.

Ain't No Mountain High Enough
– Marvin Gaye & Tammi Terrell

As the new school year commenced for 2018, I was still waiting for clearance to get back to my role at the high school, which was frustrating but understandable, given it's not every day one of your employees becomes blind.

Focusing on my swimming and the TV show, I had plenty to keep me busy. I had been in contact with the dog trainer to see where the pups were up to, to be ready for handover. Initially she told me, hopefully, there may be one suitable for me coming through in February. When I rang to find out where they were up to, she told me not many made the grade and the few that did had already been placed. I asked when the next lot would be ready and she told me most probably not until October. I was really disappointed. I guessed because the show was wanting to follow my story along with getting a dog, I didn't know what they would want to do. It seemed like it was one set back after another.

But as you will have now realised, I have always been an incredibly positive person and never one to sit back and wait for life to come along and I knew the power of *creative visualisation*. I used it plenty of times throughout my life but had just forgotten about it when I decided now was a good time to get my mind in order and start visualising the future.

Every day I would visualise sitting on the couch with Karl Stefanovic, relating how the last 12 months had unfolded. I would tell him how I went over to Melbourne to the SED training centre to get my dog. I always told him I had a wonderful time over there doing a lot of sightseeing and had a grand old time for two weeks. Even though there was no discussion or mention of the colour of dog I would eventually get, I always saw myself standing with a black dog. I would go on to tell Karl about my training regime with swimming, then I would visualise being over in Queensland swimming the races in my head. I would visualise my dive, swim the strokes and the tumble turn, then the sprint home. Always slapping the wall first, followed by receiving the gold medals on the podium. I never changed this sequence of events at all. Every day I went through the motions, emotions and excitement of getting the dog and winning the races. Over the days and weeks, I really felt like I was taking my power back and was in control of my destiny.

At the beginning of March 2018, Dee and I flew over to Sydney for the first interview with Karl for the TV show. Dee had been let into the 'cone of silence' as Hon was unable to get away from work. Dee and I kept it very low key, not telling anyone at school, while I told my mum and friends that Dee and I were just having a quick girl's weekend together. We had a fantastic little four-day holiday. We caught the red and blue line tour buses, went 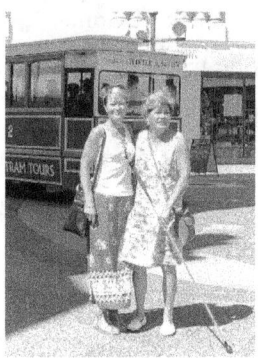 across to Manly on the ferry, did some shopping at The Rocks markets and walked about 15 kms each day. We stopped off at Bondi Beach, walked around Darling Harbour and ate at the oldest Pub in Sydney under the harbour bridge. This was special for Dee, as she reminisced about her upbringing and told me how her dad was one of the maintenance workmen on the bridge. It's lovely when you hear interesting stories like that.

I nearly fell down a manhole in the central mall in Sydney. Walking along with my pink cane, chatting away of course, when Dee grabbed my arm and stopped me. The manhole cover was up with no warning guards or witch's hats around it. Two other people also yelled at the same time seeing what was about to happen. Luckily, I was saved from what could have been a drastic mishap.

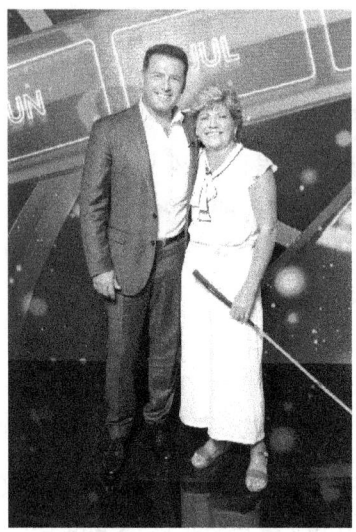

Once at the Fox studios and on the couch with Karl, I had an absolute ball. Chatting to Karl, telling my story and having some good laughs along the way. Afterwards, we were taken to the airport for our journey home with another couple who were also on the show. The studio reminded us all in the car not to divulge anything about our pledge or our story and even our driver was there to make sure we towed the line (man, that 'cone of silence' was tight). Dee and I both agreed we would forget the whole weekend and not bring it up in any conversation. That way, it would be easier to keep it secret.

Back at home, life was going along as usual when the studio was in touch again regarding the story. In the event I didn't get the dog in time, they wanted to film something I hadn't done before. With a bit of brainstorming we came up with the plan of recording my first time learning to dive into the water. I told them it was a daunting thought for me to dive into the pool, especially off a block. Not only from a vision side of things but I hadn't been able to dive for years, as the few times I had, the pain was excruciating because hitting the water ricocheted up my arm into my shoulder. If I'm to be honest, I was fearful about the pain that may very well occur, despite the fact my arms could now move freely. My recent experience was pain on hitting the water. I was scared.

The studio told me not to have any lessons until they could get a film crew to spend a day recording it.

Meanwhile, I got the all clear to start back at work at the commencement of term 2. The school was extremely accommodating and understanding as we all travelled those unchartered waters together.

While I was waiting for equipment that would help me with my job now that I couldn't see, I was given other tasks to do that didn't require special equipment.

One of these tasks was to do meditation with students who were considered at educational risk. Meditation was something I loved doing. Through Yoga, I had learned and was practicing meditation and mindfulness regularly. It's not an exaggeration to say meditation was a key coping mechanism and practice that got me through from day to day, week to week over the past year.

The students that came, after making a connection with them and chatting about what was on their mind, were keen to try meditation with me. After they finished meditating they always said they could just go to sleep and felt so relaxed and calm. It is really rewarding when you have a student come to you in tears, viewing the world well out of proportion and then after doing some positive strategies with them, have them leave with a huge smile on their face. It was always uplifting to be able to make the students feel less stressed and secure enough to connect with me, let alone the wonderful feedback from parents I sometimes received.

But being blind in the school setting did have its funny moments. I had been given quite a few new students to work with for stress and meditation. Sometimes a student would not turn up or they were a bit late. With new students whose names I had not yet learned, it was tricky to find out who was meant to be coming. So here I was, waiting in my office for the new boy to show up when a boy knocks on my door and hands me a green slip. This slip tells them who they were seeing and where to go. Of course, I can't read the form so just put it on my desk and ask him to sit down.

I introduced myself and asked him if he knew what he was here for and did he know what I did?

He answered, 'No.'

I went ahead and explained about the breathing techniques I teach to help calm you down in times of stress. Asking if he got stressed at all with school or life, he quickly responded, yes indeed, he got extremely stressed with tests and assignments. As he was late arriving to me, I asked if he would like to get straight into the meditation and next week we could have more time together. Agreeing, I put on the relaxing meditation music, went through the breathing with him followed by a visualization. We had just finished and begun talking about how he felt when there was a rapid knock on my door. Bursting open the door, Katharine said to the boy, 'What are you doing here? We've been running all around the school trying to find you. You're meant to be up getting House Captain photo's done. We sent for you half an hour ago. Quick, go now to the photo place.' Oh well, hopefully the House Captain learned some useful meditation skills. We certainly got a laugh out of that for quite some time.

To introduce myself to the new year sevens and eights I hadn't met previously, I would go into a digital-tech class and introduce myself. I gave them a short overview of what had happened to me and asked if they had any questions. There were always questions. After all, how many people know someone who has had a heart transplant or is blind? I certainly hadn't before it happened to me. The questions were always very sensible and I was open with my answers. Then I would show them how I answered the phone and used voice over to hear everything that they would usually look at. Then they all got iPads out to have a go. This was a very noisy and comical time as they listened to Siri announce the emojis.

Part of the idea of doing this was to teach the students how to communicate with a vision impaired person. I explained if they wanted to say hello to me to always say, 'Hello,' followed by announcing their name. If I looked like I didn't remember, then to say what class they were in. That way, I could connect a voice to the correct situation. It was gorgeous when some of the students came up to me and announced their name and class, followed by a descriptive dialogue of who was on duty and quite cheekily, what they were wearing, such as one male teacher wearing a woolly white jumper, looking like a polar bear. I told the student I didn't think she should tell him that, we'll keep it just between us. I walked away with a huge smile on my face.

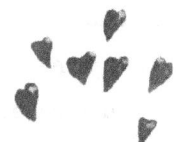

Who Let the Dogs Out
- Baha Men

While I was settling back at school, the issue of what to do with my car was in the back of my mind. I loved that car, my beautiful blue Hyundai Tucson SUV. Even though it was an inanimate object with no way of emotional expression possible from it, I knew it loved me, as I did it. I was holding on to the slimmest hope my vision may come back. Not quite ready to accept the final reality of my life 'ever after', all manner of things were getting me down. My swimming times were not improving, despite all the training and it looked like the prospect of a dog was so far 'out of sight'. Ha ha, I may as well forget it. It was a time when I really felt like I wasn't getting anywhere, where everything was hard and my life was on hold, even though I had been religiously meditating and visualising achieving all my goals. I knew there was something blocking my progress.

One Saturday morning at the beginning of April, after talking to Hon about how I was feeling, I made the decision there and then to put the car up for sale on Gumtree. Mark placed the advert on the Saturday morning and we sold it on the Sunday. The sale was smooth, easy and obviously meant to be. Both Les and I shed a few tears as the car that had helped create a lot of family memories and holidays was leaving us. It was also a symbol of my resignation of my independence, of getting around and of the permanence of my vision loss. Even though it was an emotional day, there was also a feeling of letting go of a heavy burden that had been holding me down. I felt lighter and freer within myself.

With nothing holding me down now, life could only start moving forward in a positive way. I returned to work after the April holidays and was slowly finding my feet there. Then, in the last week of May, I received a phone call from the dog trainer telling me they had a dog 99 percent ready for me. She just had to complete the final training exam and she would be mine. So excited, I asked what colour she was and was told she was black and her name was Rhian. The trainer told me she would be doing in-home training with me. This meant she would bring the dog over from Melbourne and she would be with me every day for two to three weeks while I learned how to handle the dog. Super excited, I was beaming. The trainer told me to quietly tell the school the dog could be coming within a few weeks, just to get them prepared.

Carol came in to talk to me and could see I was really excited. I told her the wonderful news, even how I had always seen a black dog in my visualisations. I went on to tell her I was a little disappointed I was having in-home training. I had been visualising flying over to Melbourne and having a grand time over there but was still extremely happy I was getting the dog.

Five weeks went by when the dog trainer called me to say she was not going to be able to do my training as she was leaving for her new job in Queensland. She didn't know if there would be delays in handing over the dog and she also didn't know what they would decide to do for training, they most probably wouldn't pay for a trainer to fly over to Western Australia to do it. Neither did she think they would have me by myself over in the training centre. Now that was all in limbo, too. I had still been continuing with my visualisation without wavering from my original plan.

Then, at end of the first week of the July school holidays, I received a call from SEDA (Seeing Eye Dogs Australia), in Melbourne. They told me they had booked my flight for Monday morning to come over to Melbourne to the training centre. You can imagine how excited I was. Thank you, universe for making things happen in such unique and miraculous ways.

Rhian and I matched up so beautifully and quickly. The trainer had never come across such a quick bond and I was doing things in the first week that most new handlers didn't attempt until the second. It was like we had been together in a previous lifetime and were now reconnected. True to my visualisation, I certainly did have a grand old time in Melbourne, catching trains, trams and buses into the city centre, having a wonderful time exploring the city.

I must say, the SEDA training centre is amazing and so well setup, from the accommodation and training delivery to the beautiful, professional staff. Truly a remarkable service. I got on so well with Maria, the gorgeous housekeeper who cooked the most amazing food for lunch and dinner. We connected beautifully, chatting together about anything and everything and are still in contact.

While in Melbourne, I met Teish Watson from Vision Australia who Siri called 'cheesy quiche'! Teish has been my navigator through all things 'support', which has made my life so much easier.

It was time to venture home after my two week stay getting to meet my new companion and soon to be best friend. When matched well, the bond between a dog and their handler is truly a deep connection,.

The trainer, Brooke, was to fly back home with me to get me settled back in the home environment and workplace, along with common places I frequented. All checked in at the airport, which Rhian skilfully led me through, we were waiting to be attended by one of the flight staff. A lovely tall man came to see what we needed to get on board easily and if there was anything we required. He was there for a minute or two and then left to get things sorted. Brooke quietly told me once he had gone that Rhian had her nose sniffing his crutch the whole time. He was so professional and polite, he never lost eye contact with either her or me, not even a twitch. We had a quiet giggle between ourselves. I was totally unaware, of course, as I couldn't see her doing it. Rhian's unsociable crutch-sniffing habit would be something that was to become a frequent occurrence and something that required some serious training.

The second night at home with Rhian was funny indeed. Our pool fence panel at one end was down while the men of the family had been cutting down a palm tree. It was pitch black outside and I let Rhian out to explore her new environment.

Les and I were chatting happily outside about my time in Melbourne when SPLASH.

'The dog's in the pool. Quick grab her, she might drown,' came the shout from Les.

The boys come running out trying to grab Rhian but every time she came close to the edge, she swam away again.

'GRAB HER. We don't want the dog to drown,' shouted Les again.

'Don't shout, you'll only make her more stressed,' I said to Les. I gently called her over to the steps and she got out of the pool and did a huge shake all over us. The rule now was not to let the dog out of the house until the pool fence was back up.

At the beach, we were to soon find out she is a real water baby and has no fear of water or waves, sticking her head under the surf to fetch a toy and will freely swim right out over the waves and surf back in with her frisbee in her mouth. A true retriever is Miss Rhian, never wanting to get out of the water. Enough is never enough for her. When we take her to the beach, onlookers are amazed by how much she loves the water. I don't think she could ever drown.

I have to say that, out of this whole process from transplant to losing vision and relearning how to do things, having a companion dog was by far the most challenging. Not only me getting used to Rhian and her settling into her new environment but also teaching the family the rules of what they can and can't do with her. Going into the school environment was a real challenge, with staff and students wanting to interact with her. I knew it was only natural but being new to me as well, it was quite a stressful time. With me still learning how to handle the dog, contending with other people made me always on edge. There were quite a few stress tears shed during those first few weeks or so. It was quite overwhelming.

I guess I imagined having a Seeing Eye Dog would be more automated or robotic, if that's the right analogy. There is certainly a lot more interaction and concentration needed when walking with her. You always have to understand the dog and what they may be feeling and be aware of the environment you are in.

In saying that, now I have had her for two years, it is so much easier as we are in sync with each other and seem to know what each other is feeling. I can't imagine life without her now. It just doesn't feel right not having my partner by my side.

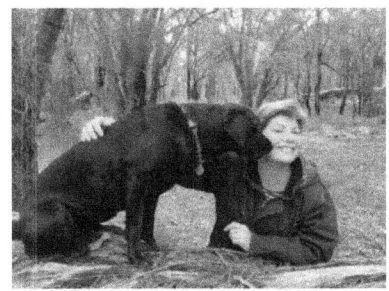

One good piece of fortune seemed to follow the next. Mark, a real motor-head, had always loved quad bikes, motor bikes and cars. As luck would have it, our new next-door neighbour, Andrew, owned a mechanic repair shop and needed an apprentice. A knock on the door with a phone number and an offer to take Mark on was received. I thanked the universe for giving him this opportunity.

Scott had been at work with a car yard for ten months but so far, had only been detailing (cleaning), the cars. He'd had very little opportunity to get into the workshop.

When Andrew came over to sort out the paperwork for Mark, Scott walked in from work and mentioned how envious of Mark he was of his apprentice opportunity. Andrew asked Scott a few questions about what he had been doing and within five minutes, both the boys were signed up to work and go through an apprenticeship together with Andrew.

Gratitude is not enough to express how we all felt about this most fortunate opportunity. We couldn't wipe the smile off Scott's face for days and Mark was excited with leaving school and going into something he was passionate about. As for me, I was relieved that universe had taken my worries about the boys' pathway into jobs that would have a future. Ask any parent of a child living with disability—their future is by far the biggest worry. Now that constant concern was taken from me, with much relief.

We Are the Champions
– Queen

Time was now marching along quickly with only three months until the Transplant Games. I had arranged to have some diving lessons but had to wait until the film crew could come out to film my efforts. In the interim and perhaps a little late in the preparation, I thought I might get some training lessons on style to try and improve my times. And so, a beautiful connection with Gemma, my swim coach, began. We hit it off straight away. I thought I was quite a good swimmer but by the time Gemma had pulled my old style apart and modified it with new techniques, I realised that techniques had certainly changed over the past 40 years. When I was relearning to swim with the new style, I felt like I was going to drown. I was like a kid learning to swim for the first time but eventually it became natural. She certainly progressed me in fitness and improved times and helped me with my mental edge.

Then it came time to record my first attempt at diving into the water. With the film crew there, Gemma started me with sitting on the pool edge and tipping forward, followed by kneeling on the side of the pool, progressing slowly to standing and rolling in. It was quite a strange feeling falling into the water not knowing when I was going to hit. Much to my relief, my shoulders didn't hurt when I broke the water. Then it was crunch time. Time to face my fears and see what I'm really made of. Standing up on the block, I had the unnerving sensation of being so high up, getting my feel of where I was standing. I seemed to wobble a little, my balance was shaky, and with arms up over my head and leaning forward all the while, the fear and dread of the pain ricocheting up through my shoulder was nagging in in my head.

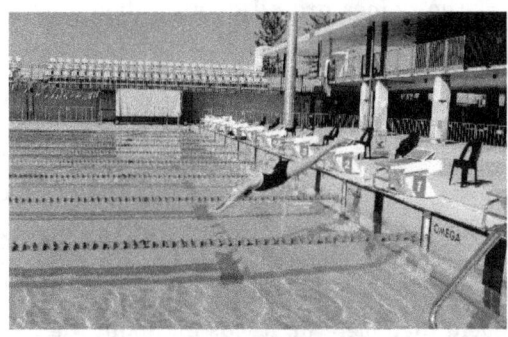

Talking me through the process as I stood up on the block, Gemma then told me to, 'Go.' Time seemed to stand still before I hit the water. It's hard to explain the sensation I felt between moving off the block and hitting the water. When I did hit the water, it was a shock. I had no idea when it was going to happen but boy was I relieved I didn't experience any pain in my shoulder and the dive was relatively smooth, except for my goggles coming down over my face. I did a few more dives, getting used to hitting the water with little warning and with practice, felt a bit more confident about successfully achieving my race dives.

I continued being coached by Gemma, who was now incorporating a proper race stance on the block. This was a little more interesting because I wobbled quite a lot; obtaining balance with a split stance is a bit tricky with no vision. Eventually, I became proficient at it. I wished now I had coaching earlier on but at least I had got a few weeks, which was better than nothing. If I was going to achieve this goal of winning gold, I wanted to do it with 100% effort.

Janine, my dear friend from school, had volunteered to be my companion to support me at the games. Les, Scott and Mark would come over after the weekend to be there for the main events. While on the plane on the flight over, I had to tell Janine about the TV show and that a film crew would be there and she may be on TV. Very excited about it all, I went on to tell her we couldn't spill the beans to anyone about the show while at the games. The 'cone of silence' was once again in operation.

We decided to have a bit of a girl's weekend together before the men arrived.

Janine's good friend Belinda flew up from Melbourne and stayed for a few days to join in and share in the fun. Rhian travelled very well and soon became familiar with her new surroundings on the Gold Coast. We met other people from Western Australia who were part of the games. It was very social, with lots of comradery and fun.

The games are all about public awareness of the Donate Life campaign, as well as everyone competing, celebrating the gift of life. The event is very emotional when it is demonstrated time and time again in every race and event, that all those competing would not be here but for the gift of life from an organ donor. The games are certainly not about the winning or the competition (although of course some of us were there for that.). It was all about the fact that all the competitors are alive, able to swim, walk, ride or compete in whatever event they were in. It was all about the incredible gift of a second chance at life.

The official parade went through the town centre, where each of the Australian states, New Zealand and Thailand walked behind their flag. We all had official state uniforms and it was quite an experience, especially for Rhian. Being in a tight crowd with a lot of noise, she walked well in the busy and crowded parade until we had to walk past the military band. The loud screeching cat-like sound from the bagpipes was just too much for her to contend with. Whether she thought it was a demon cat let out from hell, or the sheer pitch and volume, it was too much for her ears. I know not to take her to a military band again.

There were many opportunities for getting together socially with other competitors, none more so than the special beach dinner after the opening ceremony. Everyone mingled and enjoyed the dinner with music and the chance to talk to other members of our team,

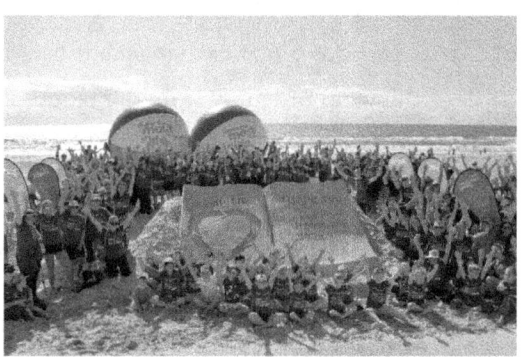

along with people from the other places. Real comradery and friendships developed in our team. The donor families also come along and enjoy the deep sense of gratitude the recipients have, all with the knowledge their loved one could be part of anyone there.

Day five of the games was my race day. The film crew had been in contact, everything was set and organised. We all arrived, Les, Scott, Mark, Janine and me. Now the nerves were starting to kick in. That annoying voice in my head, making me doubt myself about being able to achieve a gold medal.

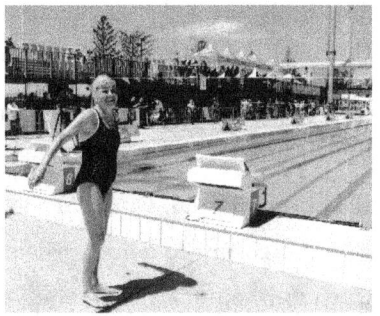

The time until my first race seemed to drag. It was as if everything was moving in slow motion and then suddenly, my first race was about to begin, the 50-metre freestyle. I very nearly missed the start as the film crew were doing a last-minute interview when Janine told me to quickly get on the block or they would start without me. This all added to the incredible build-up of nerves that seemed to overtake my body. I just made it in time to get fully into my stance before BANG, the race began. Immediately, I went into autopilot. I dived in and went full steam ahead. Focusing on nothing but hitting the wall first, I powered with all my might. In my head, I kept going through my mental reminder. Legs. Length through my arms. More legs. Legs. Length through my arms. More legs. On and on I went into the tumble turn and back into my rhythm. Legs. Length through my arms. More legs. All the time just following the long trail of the black line to finally slapping the wall to finish. I stuck my head up and asked, 'Did I win?' Janine bent over slapped my hand and told me yes, I had won gold.

Such a relief came over me. I had completed my pledge. Once out of the pool, everyone was saying how good I was and I hadn't fully understood why until I found out later I was a full seven seconds ahead of the second-place getter. Les was super pleased as he was worried about whether I would be able to pull off a gold medal, he had his doubts. Now he doesn't doubt me anymore.

My final tally results of the games were four gold medals and a silver. So, I had done what I had set out to do. Blind and with a new heart, here I was, triumphant in the pool. I had come from hardly being able to walk with my old heart, through the traumatic transformation of a transplant and all it entails, the setbacks, the hospital visits, the impact of the medication on my body, the bloody diabetes always there and always seeming to throw a spanner in the works, to realising my goal and my dream of competing and winning in the Transplant Games. I was on top of the world.

I've reflected often about whether making the pledge of winning gold for the TV show made any difference to my performance in the pool. My conclusion is that it totally did. Once I'd made the pledge and said it–said it in public–I was under pressure to achieve. I've read how important it is to make milestones and to share them with someone and now I've learned first-hand of doing the same. Yes, I gave myself additional pressure and was full of doubts and fears; doubts about my ability to win and fears around how I would feel if I didn't win. I did achieve my goal and I re-learned that valuable lesson that we can achieve anything if we put our body, mind and soul into it.

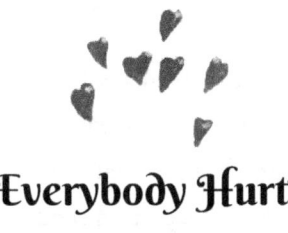

Everybody Hurts
– R.E.M.

Home from the excitement and thrill of the games, I found myself in a state I didn't understand. The last two years my life had been a constant charge forward. Finally getting listed for transplant and having all the tests and preparatory procedures to do the transplant, followed by the recovery roller-coaster-ride. I had been constantly trying to prove I could get back to normal as quickly as possible, taking on the Transplant Games, then topping it off with the TV show. Learning a new life as legally blind and getting Rhian was a bombardment of one challenge after another. These were all things I had chosen to take on willingly and with excitement. I had done it all. Proved I was a positive force to be reckoned with and anything that was thrown at me, I could take on and master. Never stopping to take a breath, there was no time for that.

Now what? What do I do next? What's my purpose in life?

I began to crumble inside. Finding myself teary and feeling very down, not quite at the stage of depression but close, I was trying to keep it all within myself as I couldn't let anyone see I wasn't coping, that just wasn't me.

There was a day when Hon picked me up just to get me out of the house after she had picked up I was struggling after a conversation we'd had. Driving in the car with her, I couldn't speak and tears just kept welling up inside me. The beauty of a true friendship is you don't have to talk all the time, it's just being there in each other's presence that matters. That's the deep connection we have with each other.

I began the process of coming to terms with the rest of my life. I started downloading motivational and positive thinking books. Even though I was familiar with most of the content I was reading from my lifelong interest in self-improvement and self-actualisation, sometimes we just have to revisit and refresh.

This set me in the right direction. I started a gratitude diary, writing in it each night even though I couldn't see what I had written. I knew it was the intention that really mattered. Focusing more intently on being mindful and present, accompanied by daily meditations, I was in a reading frenzy and couldn't devour enough of the books. I was heading in the right direction but there was something deeper that wouldn't settle inside me. Bursting into tears when I arrived on Tracy's doorstep for a Bowen session one day, she suggested I see a psychologist to delve deeper. Tracy was amazing with her therapy and I always felt better after but she knew this moment would eventually happen. She had just been waiting for things to slow down for it to register within me.

I took her advice and made an appointment with a local psychologist. Staying true to my stoic and independent private nature, I did this without telling anyone, not even my husband. I guess I saw it as I sign of weakness, I was always the strong person that got through anything. I was the pillar of strength that keeps the status quo and everybody in a safe and happy place. Why would I need mental help? Only three close friends knew and they took me to and picked me up from the sessions. Knowing I wasn't the type to share my private issues, they never divulged my secret.

I made a real connection with Jacqui, the psychologist. I felt safe opening up to her. One of the things haunting me more regularly was visions of the nightmare I experienced immediately after the transplant, popping into my head throughout the day. It was making itself present as if trying to make me acknowledge it. I thought this might have been the underlying issue.

There was also this self-awareness that I knew I wasn't smiling as much as I used to. Working that part out with Jacqui, she suggested it may be because now blind, I'm not getting the body language and subtle facial signs people are expressing and I couldn't register their emotional state and respond accordingly. I'm alright in close proximity, I can hear their voice and tone to pick up on most subtleties, particularly when I know who I'm speaking with but walking through a crowd or public area, I don't receive any feedback. It's a strange feeling. I worry that people must think I'm a grumpy or sour person and that's not an uplifting thought for your soul.

During the sessions, we revisited my nightmare using Eye Movement Desensitization and Reprocessing (EMDR), a psychotherapy treatment originally designed to alleviate the distress associated with traumatic memories. It works by helping the emotion behind a memory to become integrated by the brain. This enables you to bring up the memory without having an emotional attachment to it. I was certainly surprised at how well it worked for me. The actual session is emotionally harrowing, involving a lot of tears but the result is a positive one.

I also now understood why I had no memory of anything that happened from being told the transplant was happening straight away to waking up after the four days in the induced coma. I couldn't tell you the official terminology but it's all about the fight and flight response when you're suddenly given a huge stress response. Even though I thought I was calm and collected about it all on the outside, internally my mind had switched to full flight mode and was skyrocketing.

My flight response caused an ongoing and incomplete loop to go on in my head as I tried to recall the missing hours before the transplant and make sense of the terrible nightmare I endured while in the coma. I cannot stress how significant this nightmare was on my wellbeing each and every day, despite my best efforts of trying to push it away.

Undergoing therapy with Jacqui, I now know the reasons behind my brain and body's reactions, which has helped come to terms with my flight response and more significantly, the impact on me of my terrible nightmare. Jacqui explained I had PTSD. I am truly grateful for Jacqui helping me to understand

and sort out my mind state.

Over 12 sessions, we delved into many aspects of my life. We went back to long forgotten and sometimes painful memories to answer some of my 'why?' questions. You know the ones—the questions you don't ask yourself. Why do I feel I have to do everything myself and not ever ask for help? Why do I need to be constantly busy to feel validated? What is it about my childhood, my experiences over many years that have made me who I am today, warts and all?

Without going into the issues uncovered as a mark of respect to others who are part of my story, I can honestly say, despite the tears and at times, the great pain in exposing so many of my long-entrenched behaviours and ways of thinking and reacting, it was and still is, one of the most cathartic and healing processes I've undertaken. Having someone ask the right questions at the right time to help me heal was such an awakening for me. I really wasn't expecting such an amazing experience. I had issues that were stopping me from moving on. In fact, it's fair to say they had stopped me in my tracks.

The sessions with the psychologist awoke a hunger to know myself more fully. So, I continued on my self-development journey, going deeper into my spiritual beliefs, learning more about the universal laws, karmic patterns and the metaphysical way of life. Again, it was often revisiting a lot of the things I was interested in during my 20s and 30s before life, children and being a family became the priority.

Often, we must leave behind parts of ourselves to be able to focus on the current situation. That is a normal process of getting caught up in the treadmill of life. Then the tables turn back to another part of the circle of life and if we are lucky and aware of what's happening, as I believe I have been, we reunite with the aspects of ourselves that have been left behind or overshadowed. All through my life, I have been exposed to and interested in alternative medicine, unorthodox treatments and spiritual metaphysical beliefs. Mum had first taken me to a Chinese acupuncturist when I was 13, trying to cure my diabetes. I read a lot of astrology books and magazines through my teens and early 20s and came across my initial encounter with channelled works about the reality of life and energy that exists beyond the physical, dense world we are here to experience through this incarnation. Cassette tapes were the norm of the 80s and I would listen to the intriguing knowledge the guides were channelling through a person. Naturopaths led me to homeopaths, who I still use regularly today with great belief, knowing how amazingly it works.

I can tell some pretty amazing stories of how Scott was cured of an extremely severe stutter afflicting him at three and four years of age. His stutter was so bad, a university study I had him in told me they didn't think he would ever get rid of it completely. Finding a homeopath who went through his behaviours and gave me a remedy to give him, saw him stutter free within three days.

Mark, as a young toddler and child, suffered from asthma and allergies. Again, it was another homeopath who gave me remedies for Mark, so we were able to get him through an asthma attack just using her remedies. Now some might say it's the placebo effect but my response is, how would a four-year-old know about that?

I started going to a Kinesiologist who taught educational brain gym. I would take Stephen and Mum along in the mornings, knowing that switching on the brain and electrical circuits in the body and cross patterning was a crucial part of a child's brain development. I finished up working for her for many years. Scott and Mark would also have regular sessions with her, helping them with their learning and development.

Mum studied Reiki and Reflexology and would eventually have her own small practice with a few clients. I, for one, was a regular and still have Reiki with her. Mum has always loved crystals, too and only now am I starting to experience the beautiful energy they contain.

Thankfully, Mum was a wonderful influence along my path on the not-so-common practices, especially back then and for that, I am truly grateful to her. Don't get me wrong, western medicine is certainly vital and I wouldn't be here without it but we are more than just a physical body. The alternative or more accurately, *complimentary medicine*, treats you holistically. We are all made up of energy, meridians, auric and etheric fields. We have a spirit, mind and body, all of which need to be treated equally to maintain balance. So, it seems natural we address all these parts of our being.

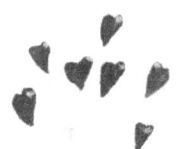

Father and Daughter
– Paul Simon

May was upon us and Dad would be 90 at the end of the month. He had become frailer and was regularly being taken by ambulance to hospital. He was diagnosed with type 1 diabetes when he was 60. He was initially diagnosed with type 2 diabetes but after a year of unsuccessful blood sugar control, I referred him to my endocrinologist. After running more blood tests, my specialist said to Dad, 'Well, I know that you're Colleen's father now, you have type 1 diabetes.' Dad always repeated this and seemed quite chuffed about the claim of belonging to me.

Dad was regularly found collapsed in his home in a diabetic coma or 'hypo' as it is commonly known by diabetics. His second wife, Ellie Mae, died two years before and he missed her terribly. She was his reason for living, looking after her with her ailments and now his reason was gone. He always expressed how he wanted to be with her again in the afterlife. It's incredibly sad when you know your parent is desperately lonely and wanting to exit this life. It becomes just one long waiting game for the inevitable to happen. How sorrowful that must be.

We decided to have his 90th Birthday at my home, we had a large patio and Dad was familiar with it. Just keeping it to the direct siblings so it was not too overwhelming for Dad, an afternoon party was arranged. It was the first time in about 20 years all of us were back together. With Geoff working FIFO, he missed Dad's 80th birthday. Will had been living up on Christmas Island for about five years, so he wasn't around either. The beauty of our family is that we may not see one another all the time but when we do catch up again, it's just like old times and great conversations are always enjoyed. There has never been any animosity in our family at all.

The day was bright and sunny, especially being one day from the start of winter. Dad caught up with all of us. Photos were taken and it was certainly a lovely reunion of our family. I quietly said to a few of my brothers that I reckon Dad will die now within the next few weeks. He had caught up with all his children and his family were all together again, his job was done and everything was OK. They agreed with my sentiments and were thinking the same thing. None of us were sad with this thought but glad he got to be with his treasured family once more before he went.

It was only a few weeks later that Dad was once again admitted to hospital. His diabetes was out of control, organs failing, along with having suffered a heart attack in that time. Within four days, Dad was finally with his beloved Ellie Mae. Finally, at peace and released from his anguished state of living. Even though it is a sad event when a loved one dies, I couldn't be sad for Dad. Knowing what his wishes were for over 18 months, it was truly a happy blessing for him. Finally, being released from his chains of living on Mother Earth.

I told David, who was arranging the funeral, that I would love to do a eulogy. He was pleased I was going to do one. He had written one focused around Dad's life and business. I decided to do one from my perspective as his daughter and the wonderful influence he had on our lives. Dad was always a very philosophical person, going with the flow of life, never getting overly excited with things that happened, good or bad. He always told me the best way of living your life was to aim to be calm and methodical. He was a wonderful influence on anyone who knew him.

The funeral was held in the country town of Northam, about 45 minutes' drive from Perth. It was the closest funeral parlour to Wongan Hills where Dad lived.

It was booked for 10 am. Stephen came and stayed overnight so we could all go together. Hon was picking up her mum and then my mum and us would follow her up.

A gorgeous day for a funeral, the sun was out and blue skies were overhead. Getting close to Northam, Stephen needed to stop at a little garage to buy some cigarettes. Telling him to wait until we got there, he replied it would only take a minute to stop and get some, so we pulled over while he ran inside and got what he needed.

Back on the road within two minutes, all was good. With Stephen chatting along merrily and Les participating in the conversation, time was flying buy. I had a little thought jump in my head telling me we should be there by now. Then Hon called to ask where we were. 'Still on the road,' was my reply.

Apprehensively, she said, 'OK. When you come over the bridge you turn right.'

Continuing along, I said to Les that we should be there by now.

'Where are we?' I asked.

Looking at the signposts along the road, he said, 'MK 15.'

'Meckering! Quick Scott, get out Google Maps and find out where we are,' I replied.

Les pulled over and started to turn back around. Scott told us we were 30 minutes away. A wave of panic and embarrassment over the thought of missing our own dad's funeral washed over us all. Les began to speed like a maniac and I told him to slow down.

We were already late. 'It doesn't matter,' I said. 'Better to be late than dead on arrival. It really doesn't matter now.'

David called and asked where we were. Meckering was my answer.

'Meckering!' He laughed and asked how we got there.

I told him Stephen was chatting the whole time and Les missed the turn off and well, here we are at Meckering. I told him to start without us, we will come in quietly through the back door.

He said, 'No, it's OK, we'll wait a bit longer. Don't stress.'

Knowing all the rest of the family and guests at the funeral will be blaming him for being late, Les was so embarrassed. I told him not to worry; we'll just make light of it.

David called again and asked how far away we were now.

'About 15 minutes,' I replied. I told him to start without us as it's getting late, especially if there is another funeral booked afterwards.

'No, don't worry we'll wait,' he answered.

'Why? Who else are you waiting for?' I asked.

'Just you,' he laughed. 'It's OK, everybody is chatting away in the funeral parlour, catching up with one another,' he calmly told me. 'We'll wait out the front for you and we can all walk in together.'

Finally arriving, David and his wife, Gail having a giggle over the morning's event put us in a lighter state of being. As I followed David and Gail down the long aisle to the front pew, I could hear a few comments about how we got lost. I stopped and brightly announced to everyone, 'Sorry for being late. It was such a beautiful day for a drive in the country and I was busy enjoying the scenery, I completely missed seeing the sign to turn off!'

People had a bit of a laugh at this and I think it lightened the mood of any impatience that may have been brewing.

It was a completely full house and ten-or-so guests had to stand at the back the whole time. I wasn't expecting such a large turnout, quite a surprise indeed.

After David and his daughter, Joanne both gave their eulogy, it was my turn. With Rhian at my side, I chose not to stand in the booth with a microphone but just projected my voice so everyone could hear. I was told later it was a beautiful speech and had brought back a lot of childhood memories for my brothers and cousins. I felt good being able to stand up in the front of a full service and proudly reminisce about Dad.

I love you, Dad.

I know you'll be having a quiet laugh about your only daughter being late for her own father's funeral.

Faith

– George Michael

It was a couple of weeks after Dad died that he came to me in a meditation. Quite often when I meditate, there is a big old oak tree with a bench seat underneath, at the top of a green hill overlooking a lake. I often sit under the oak and ask it the question, 'What do I need to know?' Then I sit and wait for whatever comes to me.

In the meditation, Dad walks up the hill toward me and then sits next to me on the bench. He tells me how happy he is being with Ellie Mae again, and everything is perfect. He never believed in an afterlife and always thought when you die your soul died too and the legacy you leave behind is in your children. Now he knows there is an afterlife and now understands how it all works.

He then told me had a gift for me and placed a pendant with a piece of golden topaz around my neck. He told me it would bring me what I needed and to use it. Standing up, he said he had to go back to Ellie Mae as she was waiting for him. I told Dad she is welcome to come up any time with him to visit. He said she was happy to wait down near the lake while he and I had time together but she knows she is welcome. Hugging each other with heart-felt warmth, I watched as he returned to his beloved Ellie Mae. Ellie Mae waved to me and smiled as I waved back.

After the meditation, I had to research what golden topaz was and what its metaphysical purpose was. I had never even heard of it. Finding out its purpose, I told Mum I needed to find a crystal place to get some golden topaz. She helped me search some places and after several phone calls inquiring about the topaz, the answers were all the same. No, we haven't had any golden topaz since the 90s, even then it was quite rare to obtain. After two weeks of searching, I gave up and thought maybe it wasn't really something I had to do. I forgot about it and carried on with my merry way of life.

Meditating once again as I did most days, Dad popped in for another visit. Walking up the hill and sitting next to me under the oak tree on my bench, he placed the golden topaz around my neck once more. He tells me it is a gift from him and I will find it and to trust my intuition. He then walked back down to Ellie Mae, who waved goodbye to me with a smile.

The July school holidays were upon us and I asked Mum if we could go down to Fremantle and try and find the golden topaz. There are lots of little, quaint unique shops there, so perhaps we would have some luck. That was the plan. Then, in a meditation the night before we were to go to Fremantle, the word 'Hillarys' flashed into my head.

Meeting Mum in the morning for our trip to Fremantle, I asked if we could go to Hillarys instead? She asked why, so I told her the word 'Hillarys' came to me in a meditation. 'I think that's where we will find the golden topaz,' I said.

'Do you know whereabouts in Hillarys?' she asked.

'No. Just Hillarys. I guess we'll find it there somewhere,' I answered.

Mum, being very intuitive and spiritual herself said, 'Well that's a good enough reason to go there for me.'

Off we went to Hillarys on a quest to find the mystical golden topaz.

Pulling into the car park and beginning to walk over, Mum said there was a crystal shop up this end of Hillarys.

'Yes, that's right,' I excitedly rejoiced, suddenly filling up with hope now.

We walked into the crystal shop, which was quite busy and hard to manoeuvre with Rhian, with the many glass cabinets and crystals everywhere. While Mum was looking at crystals she wanted for herself, the shopkeeper came over to me and asked if I needed some help. I asked her if she had some golden topaz, in pendant form. She came back straight away saying that they hadn't had golden topaz for years. It was something that was always hard to find, even back in the day when it was really popular.

'I can show you some other golden pieces like citrine that we've got,' she added helpfully.

'No, it needs to be golden topaz. I'm sure you must have it. It came to me in a meditation. I'm really disappointed now, I was so sure you would have it in a pendant,' I said despondently.

As the shopkeeper looked through the glass cabinet at the back, she squealed with disbelief. 'I don't believe it. Right at the back, there is a pendant with a piece of golden topaz on it. I didn't even know it was here.' Taking it out of the cabinet, she cheerfully bought it over to me and let me feel it.

I was so excited. Not so much about the piece of golden topaz but following my intuition and guidance through meditation, the gift Dad gave me was miraculously found.

The shopkeeper was astounded by the whole story and how I came here to find it and she still didn't know she had that piece of golden topaz.

'Certainly, something esoteric is going on for sure,' she said with a smile on her face. 'I'm so glad the piece is going to someone like you, something special has just happened.' She gave me a good discount on it as well, happy it was going to someone who knew the spiritual value of it.

It was the first time that following my spiritual guidance came through so clear and I trusted it enough to follow it. Thanks, Dad for starting me on my trusting inner guidance journey. Once you begin to follow and trust, it does become easier and things just miraculously happen, for sure.

So, for quite a while and certainly since I'd had the adrenalin rush of striving for and achieving my goals at the Transplant Games, I started delving into all sorts of self-awareness, self-fulfilment books and writings. One of these was the power of visualization and I'd like to share with you a story of this power.

One morning in January 2020, Mum and I had finished at the pool and were getting into the car. I put my phone and water bottle on the roof while I put my bag in the back. Instantly, a voice went off in my head, 'Don't put things on the roof, they'll get forgotten.' As we all do, I disregarded it, thinking I wouldn't do a stupid thing like that. Grabbing my water bottle off the roof, I sat in the car and off we drove.

As we drove along, we didn't think anything of the thud we heard, going at 100 km's an hour along the highway, all was good until we got home and I realised I'd left my phone on the roof of the car. Damn. Not letting anger or annoyance take over, I called to mind what I had been reading and believing, that everything happens in divine order and to trust the universe. Everything is as it should be.

At home, Mum suggested calling the phone company. Cutting her off, I told her, 'No, don't worry. I'll get my phone back. Trust.'

I went straight to my gratitude diary and wrote, *'I am truly grateful for me losing my phone and everything is at it should be. But I would be extremely grateful if I could have my phone back by the end of the day in perfect working order and undamaged. I totally trust this has happened for a reason and I'm OK with that but I would really appreciate it if I can have my phone back. Everything is as it should be. Thank you.'*

Closing it up and putting it away, I put my workout shoes on, set up my weights, started playing some uplifting workout music and began my resistance training.

20 minutes later, Mum came down and said, 'Do you want a surprise?' Looking at her, I said, 'Was it in the car?'

The thud we heard was the phone going off the back window of the car. The phone fell on the side of the highway. As fate would have it, that day, and only that one day of the year, a maintenance crew were working to clean up and mow the side of the road exactly where my phone landed.

One worker was on the ride-on mower while the other was on the verge. As the mower was moving forward, the sun glinted on the phone screen and the other worker saw it. Stopping the mower from destroying it, he picked it up. As he had it in his hands, Les called. The man answered the phone and Les says, 'This is my wife's phone.'

The man told him he had just found it on the side of the highway. He told Les it was lucky he called when he did, otherwise he wouldn't be able to unlock the phone to find out who it belonged to. He continued that if it were any other day, it would not have been found as it would be another year until a maintenance crew came along this stretch of highway.

So, I got my trusty phone back, in perfect working order and luckily, completely undamaged. I immediately went back into my diary and wrote, *'Thank you. I am truly grateful for getting my phone back so quickly and undamaged. That was certainly impressive work there, universe. Thank you and everything is as it should be.'*

That was a very self-affirming confirmation, that the words and thoughts we put out there certainly do have a lot of influence and power. If I had said, 'I've lost my phone. It's going to cost me a fortune to get another. How am I going to get everything back on it?' etc. that's exactly what would have happened. You really must be positive and know exactly what you are thinking and saying all the time. It's all energy and way beyond our comprehension. I guess that's why we have those old sayings like, 'Careful what you ask for,' and, 'Ask and you shall receive.'

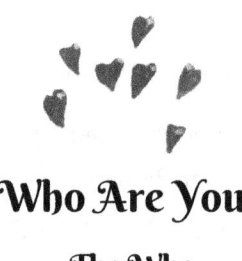

Who Are You
– The Who

Back at school in term 3, and secretly awaiting the exciting finale of going back to Sydney for the final filming of the TV show. Keeping this secret was quite a task, especially since Mum lives on the same property as us and has always been on our family holidays with us. It was no easy task but with time spent getting our stories straight and having to invent a reason for why we were going over to Sydney, we managed to pull it off.

We enjoyed a lovely family holiday and Stephen also came along because the show wanted him in the audience. Let alone having all of us back together on vacation, we all had a ball filming the last part of the story. Rhian also got to be a star as she walked out on to the stage and lay there looking her normal gorgeous, sleek and glossy self. I was really pleased I got the opportunity to experience something like that. It is certainly an eye opener to know how shows are put together and the amount of time and filming goes into what ends up as such a short amount of viewing time.

I had joined my local branch of Toastmasters some time before going on TV, simply because I wanted to make sure I had the confidence to speak in front of an audience and with the host of the show, Karl. Quite aside from really enjoying the whole Toastmasters experience and the great people I met there, it really gave me the 'I've got this' feeling, so I was confident and relaxed when it came to recording the show. More than that, I LOVED being in front of an audience and being in the spotlight.

Back home and back to business as usual and still sworn to secrecy but before long, commercials started appearing on TV about the show. I hadn't even seen one when I began receiving text messages from friends saying they saw me on TV. Still not being able to say what it was about, excitement was starting to buzz again.

It was another four or five weeks before my episode was to be aired. Sitting together as a family to watch it was the plan. However, the universe in its weird and wonderful way of orchestrating things, had another idea. I had been having issues the previous few weeks with shortness of breath and the muscles in my legs seizing up while walking to work, to the point I couldn't do it anymore. So, a hospital stay was the hand of cards dealt to me instead of enjoying my TV debut with my family on the couch at home. I couldn't believe the odds. How uncanny can timing be? I guess the universe thought being back where it all began was quite appropriate, in a weird sort of way.

The staff on the CCU all knew me from my previous stays and word had got around I was on the show that night. The nurses had even shared it with great pride on the hospital Facebook page. Les had worked a long day, plus he had an early start in the morning, so I told him not to worry about coming in. It didn't really bother me so long as I got to see it, that's all that mattered. Eddie phoned to see if Les was coming in to watch it with me. When I explained about the work situation, he told me he would drive down straight away to watch it with me. He is the most caring and protective brother anyone could ask for; he always comes running to my side if he thinks I need it.

I received text messages from friends as soon as the show had finished and it was certainly an ego booster. I had a smile on my face as I read them all. The following morning, the team came around and I received more accolades. They were extremely proud of me and my performance. They were pleased with how it came across because it was a really positive promotion for transplants. Positive vibes were bouncing all around the ward that day. I even had a stranger, who I met when I was going down the lifts with Rhian and Les the next day, say they saw me on the show and how inspirational I was. Now try and wipe that smile of my face, let alone fit my head through the lift doors, and they are really wide.

Arriving at school the following week, further adulations were received. The school had also shared it on their Facebook page. Some of the students came up to me asking if I was a television star. I told them, 'No. Far from it but thanks for thinking of me as one.' I felt like the school hero as well.

Here Comes the Sun
- The Beatles

Life returned to normal. Nothing further exciting was to come or was planned. I was just in the normal rhythm of everyday living. I was beginning to enjoy a slower pace. Les may not agree with that statement as my schedule hadn't really changed, except I wasn't pushing myself in the pool. Swimming three days a week, Pilates and yoga. Dancing one night a week and Toastmaster's once a fortnight, along with still walking to school each morning, was enough to keep me going.

As the new decade of 2020 clicked over, my main attention over the past few months was with pursuing my spiritual awareness. I had a real yearning to know and understand myself at a deeper level. I had always been focused on the physical aspect of life. Always powering along in energy, often to the detriment of my body. Never stopping to be still and to listen to my body. Yoga had been a huge benefit for me, I had gradually learned to slow down, breathe and have compassion for myself and my body.

Continuing with my reading, practicing meditation every day and having an awareness of the trees, birds and just everything surrounding me, I was always in awe of just how amazing Mother Earth really is.

On my walk to school there were three special trees I passed and I called them 'The Sentinels'. I could feel their presence as I walked by and I said, 'Good morning,' to them each time, acknowledging the true spiritual energy within them. Tuning in to the trees, I could feel their energy and was constantly grateful for everything in my life. Life had been and was still flowing so smoothly, I loved and accepted everything that entered my reality. The one thing I had come to accept is, we are exactly in life where we are meant to be.

Despite all this, the one thought that was constantly in my head was, 'What is my life's purpose?' I know everyone must think that, too but this was consuming my soul. The deeper I delved into study and myself, the more hauntingly the question echoed in my head.

Two weeks into the school year and we were hearing about the Corona Virus or COVID-19. Life still cruised along as normal but announcements on the radio and news were telling of more cases around the world. It still seemed to be 'out there' and we here in Australia were thinking how lucky we were to not have any here. Of course, that illusion was soon to be shattered as the days went by.

Things started to change with increasing restrictions being announced daily. Not surprisingly, being 'high risk', I was sent home from school to keep out of danger. Confinement at home was something I had been used to but this was different. For some reason, this lockdown gave me the permission I had needed to finally slow down and to take some time out. Perhaps because everyone else was doing the same and there was no guilt associated with not being busier than a blue-arsed fly at a BBQ.

With nowhere to go and no one to see, inward reflection was definitely on the menu at café universe. I personally believe this whole COVID-19 pandemic was Mother Earth's way of making us go to our rooms to sit down and reflect on how we have treated her. She has given us all time to sit back and review our lives; to think of what is important to us and re-prioritise what we value most in our life. For some, it was an opportunity to rekindle relationships with children and family and get back to the basics of life as a simple community. For me, COVID-19 gave me the chance and the time to reflect inwards and find the real me, the one that's behind the crazy, action-packed Colleen and the one who values her spiritual self.

Turn! Turn! Turn!
– The Byrds

It was during the school holidays when the idea came to me to start writing my story. I still had friends saying I needed to do it but there was always some sort of distraction I used as an excuse not to start. I had been at home for a month now and returning to school was still quite a while away, so I opened my laptop and began writing.

During this time off work, I had been continuously working on unpeeling the layers of the onion skin of self. I knew astrologically, this year especially was one of great change both personally and globally. I wanted to do everything I could to make the most out of the positive opportunities the universe presented me with.

I realised this time off work would enable me to start writing my book. The next lesson or opportunity to learn and grow was just around the corner. This corner was a sharp turn and there was no way of being able to see around it until you had already taken it.

This was a time of me becoming emotionally vulnerable. Vulnerability was one strength I had never experienced before. I had always kept myself together and very closed inside. I built huge walls over the years to keep my emotions from escaping. Now they were well-and-truly breaking down the walls to make themselves felt and integrated within me.

Ever since I lost my sight, deep-down I always felt I was destined for a different or greater journey. I didn't know what that journey would look like but I knew it wasn't working at the school. Don't get me wrong, I did love working at the school with all the students I helped and mentored. School had been more than accommodating, making whatever adjustments I required to feel comfortable at work but that feeling of fulfilment and deep satisfaction was now missing.

Each time I could have returned to work during the pandemic, I had a choice of taking another two weeks sick leave. And each time I took it, knowing deep down I didn't really want to return. Now crunch time was closing in on me and I knew I would soon be out of excuses. My body also began telling me I had to honour myself to embark upon a new journey. I knew I couldn't start my new beginnings until I had closed the door on the old but how could I just say I didn't want to go back? How could I just throw it all away knowing once that door was shut, there was no opening it again? Those were the constant questions rattling around in my brain.

My once peaceful sleeping habits began to disappear. My daily walk with Rhian became hard with shortness of breath and intense muscles fatigue. My heart started ramping up arrhythmia's and my blood pressure started to drop and fluctuate. At the time, I never associated it with the issue of going back to school. I didn't think the other stresses would have caused it, either. I was still asleep as to what the real issue was.

I managed to get the last few weeks off from going back to school because I was going back and forth to the transplant clinic. I had an event monitor which picked up the arrhythmias, which were really making me feel awful, along with my blood pressure dropping to 80/50. An echo was done and some noticeable differences were seen, so a biopsy and right heart catheter pressure test was done at the same time. A stiff heart was found, which can be a sign of rejection. However, thankfully the biopsy found none. My symptoms were getting worse until the Sunday morning just before the school holidays were about to begin, I felt really unwell. I rang the hospital and they told me to come in.

Back in hospital, I was constantly monitored, bloods taken each day and tested for all sorts of things. Lungs checked with radioactive gases and tracers to see how well the lungs were exchanging the blood gases. An exercise echo was performed and even though I couldn't complete the test because of shortness of breath and fatigue in my leg muscles, it was clear as well. Eventually, medications were added and then taken away and my heart thankfully stabilised.

For many people, going to hospital is a once or twice in a lifetime event or a rare event, in any case. For me and for other transplant recipients, it's part of life and I know I took this part of my life in my stride. No doubt all my previous health issues and hospital visits helped with my familiarity with hospitals.

Having said all that, transplants are the next level and I think, for me at least, I developed a relationship of total trust and dependency on the medical staff and teams. It comes from knowing they have taken out my heart, my life-giving pump, and given me a new one, keeping me alive all the while. It's a big deal. With that amount of time, talent, knowledge and interest they have invested in me doing well, I have felt at times as if they were in control of my body and Colleen, the person inside that body, was swept along for the ride.

Here I was back in hospital, not sure what my heart was doing, although I feel that stress (as well as the medications I was on, as it turns out) was playing a part.

As the days went by, I became doubtful about everything I had been experiencing. I knew how terrible I had been feeling over the past few weeks, along with some bad headaches, too. Then one afternoon, when I was at the hospital still undergoing tests, I texted Clare, who had told me if ever I wanted a chat to just ask and she would come up. I messaged her and she told me she would come up in an hour. I had, for most of that day, felt like bursting into tears for no reason and I didn't know what to do. I only knew I had to talk to someone and Clare had always been there for me when I was in hospital.

Waiting for Clare to come up, I tried to keep my mind on listening to an audio book. Then she came in, initially talking about the test and their findings when I told her that it's not what I'm worried about. Then the flood gates opened and they were not going to shut. I poured out my heart with everything I had been going through with Stephen and his battle with addiction. Then how I was feeling about work at school and my personal self-fulfilment level just not being there. I confided I was only just keeping my head above water and could not deal with anybody's shit (pardon my language). I couldn't face or talk to anyone and the thought of going back to school was just too overwhelming. I was tired and just wanted to stay home and lead a quiet life with no big goals to reach. I just couldn't do it anymore. I felt so frail.

Clare was truly amazing in just listening and then reflecting it back to me. She told me the team are always amazed by the things I do, how I just keep going in such a positive way and don't think any more about it. 'It's Colleen, that's what she does. But at what price?' Clare said. She told me I was her inspiration and often told other patients about me without using my name but she had no idea about everything I had been dealing with, either. She told me that right from day one, I had been on a constant drive forward, taking on one goal after another and achieving them, never having time to stop and slow down and acknowledge what I've been through.

Clare suggested that if I didn't know what makes me happy, I should at least stop doing the things that make me unhappy. 'That, to me, is giving up work.' she added. 'Take time out to just sit back and enjoy your second chance at life for a while. Let yourself have time to really recoup without the stress of thinking about going back to work. This is your time now.'

That was a life changing conversation and a time of self-realisation of what I really needed to do.

The next morning, Clare bought me in an angel pin to remind me there is always someone looking over me. I have that pin sitting on my dressing table and every morning I rub it and thank Clare for that timely and life changing conversation she had with me. People certainly do come into your life when you need them the most. For that, I will always be grateful to Clare.

I now had in my head what I had to do to move forward along my true pathway in life but there was so much uncertainty of letting go of the familiar and the feeling of security the school held for me. Honestly, I was worried how Les would react but of course I had nothing to worry about, Les was wonderful. Completely understanding, he had no issues over me leaving work at all. He just wanted me to be happy and well. He couldn't imagine a life without me in it and if I would be happier and healthier being at home, then that's what would happen. He couldn't believe I would be worried about bringing it up with him. He has always done everything to make me happy and I know that.

Resigning from work felt like a huge burden was lifted from my shoulders. Now I could move on to the next part of my soul's journey. Life without work has enabled me to continue in earnest with my self-discovery.

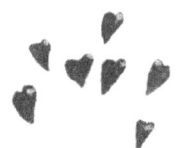

I Say a Little Prayer
– Dionne Warwick

When I woke up blind after my transplant, I started an unwinnable fight for life to return to normal. Every action and thought were, in retrospect, directed at achieving what was not possible. Things were never going to be the same. Now, given what I am learning about myself, I'm OK with that. It took an enormous amount of furious energy proving to the world I could do anything. I was just the same, if not a better (bionic), version of Colleen. Then it all came crashing down after I'd achieved my goal of winning gold at the Transplant Games and no longer had something where I could direct all my furious energy.

What is becoming apparent to me is, by not truly accepting my diabetes as a child, I closed my heart off to the disease and the impact it was having on my body and brushed it off as 'nothing special' and 'nothing to acknowledge'. What I didn't realise, I was adopting this same attitude to all the other emotional issues that came along throughout my life. Diagnosed with diabetes as a child set me up to be 'strong' and 'independent' and from an early age, I became very good at shutting down my emotional responses beyond, 'I'm alright, I don't need help.'

Anything that didn't feel right or wasn't right for me, I internalised and buried deep down. So for me, it took a heart transplant and the rollercoaster ride after this transformational event, to awaken some of the things buried deep within me. Things that needed to be addressed and resolved so I could move on.

I've never been someone who cries easily. Now, when my eyes start to water or I feel that rising uncomfortable feeling inside me, I sit with the feeling and try and sense where it is sitting in my body and ask myself, 'What is it that I am feeling? What is it saying to me?' The more I've done this and been present in these feelings and acknowledged them, the more their power over me dissipates. It's as if they are simply being asked to be acknowledged and recognised. This has taken a conscious effort as my knee-jerk reaction is still to shut them down.

I'm also learning I don't have to know everything, that I can accept help and I don't have to always be strong and take care of everyone. I know I am the sort of person who generally has it all together all the time but sometimes when I get to a speed bump, I now know it's OK to share and talk about it with someone. I've realised sharing your thoughts does not only halve them but usually resolves them as well.

I know this is a journey and my old habits are dying hard. My first response in any situation is always my old way of reacting; impatient and quick to become frustrated. Now I'm conscious of what I need to do. I will ask for help and graciously accept it when it's offered. I will sit with my feelings and give myself time to come to an understanding of where the feeling comes from and what they are saying to me.

Losing my sight has brought me to a point of quiet surrender from having to be strong, looking after everyone and accepting help for myself. My relationship with my husband has grown deeper and I can't express how grateful I am in having him as such a devoted and loving partner in life. My relationship with Mum has also grown stronger, especially over the past twelve months since we've re-embarked on our spiritual journey together after all these years. I have come to see Mum in a different light and am enjoying this beautiful connection we now have.

Instead of always being in a state of trying to work things out and thinking of what I want in life, instructed by my historic belief patterns, I now come from of a place of not having to know, spending time sitting and going within and following the breath and inner peace and truth resounding inside of me. I believe it is then that we can find out what it is we truly desire, from a higher place and not a place of ego. By not trying to work out how things are going to happen but just visualising the result and making clear, defined choices every day, serendipitous things happen in the most amazing ways.

After the transplant, people asked me if I was going to sue the hospital for what had happened and losing my sight. My initial response on hearing this was one of disbelief and bewilderment. How could anyone even think that way with how well I have recovered and why would they think I would want to? I went into this journey fully aware of the possible dire outcomes and that my chance of surviving the surgery was extremely low. If I did survive, my longevity after surgery would still be limited. The team advised against it all the way except for Dr A but all knew I took personal responsibility for my decision to continue on that path.

I have never regretted for one day embarking on such a challenging journey. Against all odds, I did survive and nearly four years on, I'm doing extremely well. Even though I lost all but a fraction of my sight, I have always recognised it as a gift to be unwrapped slowly to find the wonderful present bestowed within. I have really got to know and understand myself deeper than ever before.

I believe I was the first type 1 diabetic to ever have a heart transplant here in Perth and I would never do anything to jeopardise any other diabetics from having the opportunity I was given. We all need to take personal responsibility for our own decisions and life. There are no guarantees everything is going to turn out the way we want. If you want to ensure that nothing bad is going to happen to you, then you will never take any risks and will never find out what wonderful opportunities may be in store.

I took that risk and even though it wasn't the outcome I was expecting, I now see it as something even better. My life just didn't continue its usual familiar pattern. It has given me a much richer, deeper and new way of living, far beyond what I was experiencing before. By stepping out of your comfort zone and challenging yourself in new ways, you get to find out what you're really capable of. Blaming another person for something that happened to you is never going to solve the problem. Nobody ever wins from conflict or blame.

When people asked me what the main thing I missed with losing my sight was, my answer was always playing Canasta. Hon and I would spend most of our time together playing Canasta, progressing to Samba. For those who don't know what these games are, they're card games. Canasta uses two packs and Samba three. They are games of strategy, usually causing a medical condition resembling Tourette's. It was a huge part of our socialising. Both Hon and I were missing this aspect of our shared joy. We had tried to play with large playing cards but it was still too hard and extremely tiring for me trying to read them. We put them away and forgot about them until about a year later.

Sitting together one day and trying to work out how we could make it possible to be able to return to our shared joy, with a bit of brainstorming and Hon's ingenious idea, we soon invented our version of Blind Canasta. A combination of both Samba and Canasta, reducing the range of cards used, we are now extremely happy swearing at each other, always laughing.

After everything I have been through in my life, coming to the point I am now, the most empowering aspect I have learned is to 'know thy self'. I have filled my life with knowledge of how life seemingly works and what I believe but the point of personal power is coming to understand yourself deeply. I genuinely believe we must question why we do the things we do; we must challenge our personal beliefs and check they are truly ours and not our parent's, society's, culture, educational system or any other part of our life. Our life should be an open book, allowing not only us but others to enquire and question where we are coming from. We need to regularly check in on our reactions and learn why we react as we do, so we can move to a place of contentment, happiness and peace. None of us can create our best life if we hide, suppress or ignore aspects of ourselves that are not genuine, not authentic.

It is not a quick fix project or a couple of sessions in self-understanding but an ongoing journey for the rest of one's life. You can't create a future until you understand why it is you are wanting to create it. It is only once you realise the part of your 'self' that needs to be recognised, that you come to a point of inner peace and fulfilment.

One of the things my friends Deb and Hon have really enjoyed is that I now have, what they call 'leaky eyes'. I now cry more than I have ever done before. Both like seeing this more vulnerable side of me. Not so tough, a little more human, softer and perhaps even someone a little easier to relate to, knowing I *do* feel emotions. Hon tells me leaky eyes are just a way of cleaning the windows to the soul, so you can see the truth more clearly. I am slowly getting used to regularly cleaning my soul's windows, they are shiny and bright now and I am grateful for feeling my emotions. Now I must learn what the emotions are that I am experiencing and with time, I'm sure I will become quite proficient with them. A deep sense of gratitude goes to Deb and Hon who have really been my soul sisters, journeying together in life. I love you girls.

My one wish for everyone is to take time to discover and understand your real inner self. Then your true-life passion and path can come to be fully embraced, living a life with joy and doing the little things that bring you happiness. I believe we are here on this journey to learn who we are. Don't take things too seriously, though, and always have fun and a light heart in whatever endeavour you undertake. Remember too, everyone else is trying to work their own stuff out, so have a little compassion and understanding towards them. My true love goes out to all sharing this life on earth with me and my wish for everyone is to know there is another way of living life; one that brings peace and joy.

PS – I Love You

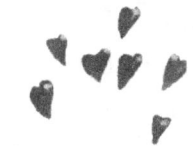

We Are Family
– Sister Sledge

I am the person I am today because of my family and those who I have had the good fortune and good sense to have as my friends. Thinking of all these important people at the centre of my life, I am blessed beyond measure. I know now, I would not have been able to do this journey alone and the team were right in saying I needed support on my transplant journey. I know my successful recovery and the rich and rewarding life I am living is due almost entirely to this unwavering and unconditional support and love from friends and family.

My dearest Les. It's difficult to put into words my feelings of love and gratitude for your unconditional love and support in everything I have done, including my crazy levels of energy and activity.

I know Les loves me at such a deep and profound level. The best way I can describe it is that he treats me like a queen. I'm truly so lucky to have such love. At times, I have felt unworthy of Les's all-encompassing love but I have come to realise the love bestowed upon me reflects the love I give out and so now accept it with great and humble gratitude.

Thank you, Les, for being such a wonderful and supportive husband and father and a caring, funny and kind partner in life. You help make my life interesting and fun with your quirky, humorous antics. You pick me up when I am down. I am truly lucky to have found you in that TV repair shop 24 years ago.

I feel so blessed to have my wonderful boys, Stephen, Scott and Mark. They have been the centre of my life and my being. A strong family life has always been my main goal and my focus and I am full of love and gratitude for my family and the journey we are taking together. I am so proud of you Stephen, Scott and Mark, you make my life richer and fuller by being in it. Thank you.

I must express how grateful and blessed I am to have married two good-hearted and loving men. Even though my marriage with Paul ended in dissolution, we have always remained connected at a heart level. Paul has looked after Stephen and me and we have maintained good communication and a good relationship. Even today, Paul and I continue to have Stephen at the forefront of our combined energies and concern and he continues to be a welcome visitor to our home. I know Paul still has a deep connection with me and I with him, at a certain level. Let's face it, once you have been committed to each other and had a child you are bound karmically for life. Thank you, Paul for sharing part of your life with me and being a steadfast and solid support for me and Stephen throughout our lives, always making sure we never went without.

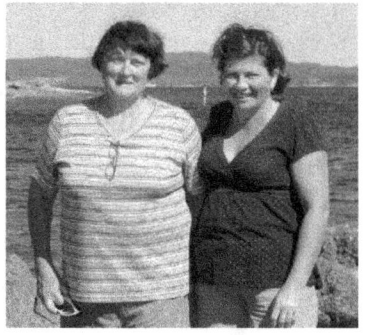

Mum. What a mother. Mum has always been by my side my whole life and even now, she is there for me, taking me to the pool so I can do my swimming, driving me to the river so I can walk along it with Rhian. Mum has always supported me in endeavours and dreams. Thank you, Mum, for truly being the most loving and caring Mum in the universe.

Eddie, my brother. I've become aware while writing this book of how, through good times and bad, you and I have stuck together. From children moving in with Mum together, to you being best mates with Paul. We have been tightly entwined all my life, never straying far from where I am. We definitely have a deep Karmic connection. Thank you for being a constant in my life's journey, always there as a protector by my side. I always know you have my back. We seem to be bound by a heart connection with each other in this lifetime and I'm sure, beyond.

Kim and Geoff had problems with addiction early on in their lives. I don't think any of us are blessed with having unscathed, perfect lives; we all mess up to some degree or another, don't we? I'm pleased to say, it was a short stage for them both. My dear brothers are married, have children and both lead successful lives.

Hon. My dear cousin and best friend. Together since we were young girls sharing our lives so closely. Old time dances with our parents, me teaching you to ride my pony Rocky, our holiday adventures together from childhood into adulthood. We have always loved our time with each other.

I want to thank you, Hon, for being in my life in our younger days and then returning after being away for a decade. When you re-entered my life with Stephen, you bought a fresh and fun energy which lifted my heart. We have kept that beautiful energy and synchronicity ever since. We know each other better than we know ourselves and can honestly and openly tell each other the truth. That is a rare gift indeed and I am so grateful, Hon, for our lives being entwined. We are connected on another level and are wonderful teachers for one another. I love any time we share together. Thank you.

While I was dealing with everything and working my way through my emotional land slide, Deb had always been there for me. In fact, ever since the transplant, Deb has made Thursday 'Coll's day'. Initially taking me to any appointments I needed to go to, then including coffees, lunches out, swimming, anything I wanted or needed to do. Deb was there when I dragged her out of bed at 6 am in the morning twice a week because I wanted to do some functional *high intensity interval training* (HIIT) training. When I said I wanted to go dancing, Deb found a new dance class in Kalamunda on a Monday night and true to being Deb, took me there and participated as well. We enjoy spiritual and metaphysical discussions and talking through a range of topics which is truly refreshing, having someone you can talk to on subjects you both find interesting and stimulating.

There are so many other friends who have been there for me before, during and after the transplant, including Sue, Shelley, Amanda and Paul, Carol and Ally and so many more. While not everyone is mentioned by name, please know your friendship and love has sustained me and I am richer for having you in my life. Thank you.

Acknowledgements

Thank You for the Music
– ABBA

I can't finish this book without acknowledging some very key people on my journey so far.

First and foremost, a deep sense of gratitude goes to the wonderful Transplant Team at Fiona Stanley Hospital. Without them, I undoubtedly would not be here today enjoying not only my dear friends' company but seeing and sharing my sons' lives. I can't imagine how much their lives would have changed through me dying. The team, including everyone I've met at Fiona Stanley have become like a second family to me as they have journeyed with me on this ride of a lifetime.

A special thanks goes to Dr Amit Shah, who recognised something in me worth fighting for, week after week. I know now the rest of the team see that special spark in me now but Dr A, you realised it first and thought I was worth fighting for. My life is indebted to you.

Nurse Practitioner Clare Fazackerley, mentioned so often in this book, has become a very special person with whom I hold a deep resonant connection.

Clare, you have always been there and intuitively seeming to know when things weren't going right. I seemed to always receive a text from you just when I needed it. Through the transplant and at other times of need, you have always been there listening to me and reassuring me. Thank you, Clare, you are a special person.

I'm not able to name all who gave me such special care during my time in the ICU and CCU but please know, you all have my sincere gratitude. I do want to mention Dr Lawrence Dembo, Mr Chris Merry and Mr Robert Larbalestier aka the 'grumpy old witchdoctor'. With all my heart, thank you.

I must mention a dear person I was introduced to when I was 18. Dr Kim Stanton, my endocrinologist, who has looked after my diabetes through all my travels over the years, all my pregnancies and travelled my life's path with me, always keeping my health at the forefront. He is a person I trust and have enjoyed many conversations with. Thank you, Kim, for over 30 years of care and being together. You will always be remembered fondly in my heart(s).

Without Tracy doing her magical Bowen and ITA energy work and Raelene supporting me with acupuncture, emotional coding and TFT therapy, I certainly wouldn't be at the point I am in my journey now. Penny, my long-term homeopath, has always been an ongoing and very important part of my health maintenance regime and knows exactly what's going on in my body to help remedy it. I want to thank these three incredibly special women who each have amazing modalities in treating the body, mind and spirit on a whole other realm.

My workplace colleagues at Lesmurdie High School quickly became my closest friends. Katharine or Sensei, as I came to call her, entered my life to have a special, deep connection of rare understanding and wisdom. A sense of confidentiality and reason was a deep connection between us. Jane and Dee, aka 'Trinny and Susannah' were the bubbles and popping corks that enthusiastically always lifted, not only mine but anyone's heart in close proximity. Light and fun but always there to back you up when things got down. Thank you, girls, for keeping me in trendy fashion and up with the latest both before and after transplant. The three of you are my 'go to' whenever I need some fun time or friends to sound off with. I know you are only one text message away and you are there for me, as I am for you.

Janine and Heather, we share a close circle of friendship and deep comradery. Janine, always excitedly ready to get on board with a mission and supporting me through the Transplant Games and anything else I was doing. Heather, not only her talents as a hairdresser but as an artist, creates wonder and a beautiful energy that anyone loves to be around. Heather not only created beautiful art for my home, she created the amazing artwork for the cover of this book. I love my time with both of you girls and thank you for all your love and friendship.

Ally, a wonderful teacher and friend got me back into dancing—rock n' roll—you made a great jive partner, thank you for all the dance moves, karaoke and girl's nights.

I would also like to thank Manny (AKA Emanuel). Manny has been my tutor since I began back at the high school after the transplant. He has very patiently endured over 60 hours of IT training with me, all the time making me feel like I'm clever and doing just great. I know some days I definitely wasn't and my brain just didn't want to retain any information but Manny remained funny, patient and very encouraging. We have got to know each other at a much more personal level and without Manny's tutoring, I most probably would not have been able to write this book. Thank you, Manny, for your patience, support and encouragement and the wonderful friendship we have fostered along the way. I just want to add that Manny is totally blind and amazed me with how efficiently and quickly he can manoeuvre through the computer. Perhaps one day I'll be half as good as Manny.

A serendipitous sense of gratitude goes to Mary-Anne, who through the weird and wonderful way of the universe randomly entered back into my life after 18 years. Mary-Anne's son, Magnus and my Stephen were great buddies in primary school. I was part way through writing this book when I said to Mum that I would need to find someone to help correct the spelling and grammatical errors. I left it to the universe find them. Then one day, in a local pet shop, after I had finished my first draft of the book, I heard a voice from the past. Excitedly saying our names, it was like we had seen each other only a few weeks before. Agreeing to catch-up in a few weeks, we exchanged phone numbers and parted. As I walked out of the shop, I said to Mum that Mary-Anne was the one who was going to help me with my book and with that, I thanked universe for that gift.

Sure enough, about six weeks later, Mary-Anne came around to my place for a catch up after 18 years of not seeing one another. Then, telling her about my endeavour of writing a book and the difficulty I was having with trying to correct it, she gleefully and excitedly said she would love to help and had the knowledge to do it. With that, Mary-Anne helped a great deal and I definitely couldn't have done it without you. Thank you.

I must, of course, give a thank you to the lovely Claudette Pope, Editor at Footprints Publishing and Co-Director, Lisa Wolstenholme. Not having any idea how to get my book published, Mary-Anne searched the web and again, thanks to serendipity, she found Footprints Publishing who publish heartfelt stories. A few clicks later, then an email, Claudette wrote back saying it would be an honour to publish my book. Claudette has been such a wonderful, funny and inspiring person to work with. Lisa has been truly creative with her design layout and presentation skills. These two remarkable, down-to-earth and very personable women have been a pleasure and joy to work with.

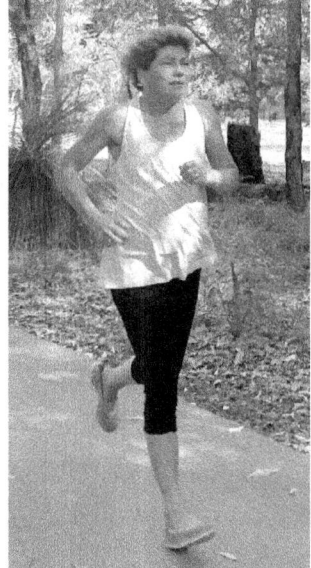

I have saved my most important and heartfelt gratitude until last. To the wonderful donor family, whoever and wherever you are. It is through this most selfless and loving gift, given in a time of great distress and grief for your loved one, that you have given the gift of life to me, a stranger. Words are difficult and certainly, there are no words that come even close to expressing the gratitude I feel for you. Thank you for entrusting me with this precious gift and thank you for a second chance of life.

Finale

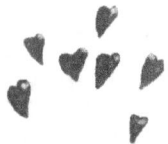

What a Wonderful World
– Louis Armstrong

Obviously, music is a huge part of my life. From my teenage years, the years of ballroom dancing and as an aerobics and Zumba instructor, music has been the ever-present golden thread so important to me on my life journey. It has provided me with joy and comfort every day. I cannot finish this memoir without providing you all with a final soundtrack that is for me, the perfect song to sum up how I feel about the world and my fellow travellers. I hope it's the same for you.

Queue 'What a Wonderful World' by Louis Armstrong.

Colleen Ashby

March 20, 2021

Author Bio

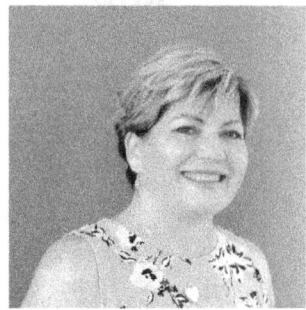

Colleen lives in the Perth Hills, in Western Australia. A former high school special-needs educational assistant and fitness instructor; she is also a type 1 diabetic.

With her heart failing, Colleen was finally put on the transplant list and had a heart transplant in January 2017. It wasn't something normally offered to type 1 diabetics. While she gained a new heart, Colleen lost 95% of her sight. This hasn't stopped her indomitable spirit or living life to its fullest.

She is an advocate for DonateLife WA, has been a 'poster-girl' for Vision Australia, a participant in the Transplant Games and a supporter of Transplant Australia.

Colleen is sharing her story of resilience in the hope it will help, inspire and encourage people to appreciate what they have and what they can achieve.

Her journey continues. With her experience, knowledge and zest for life, Colleen wants to be a mentor and motivational speaker.

Follow her on her travels at:

https://info3359876.wixsite.com/colleen-ashby

www.ingramcontent.com/pod-product-compliance
Lightning Source LLC
Chambersburg PA
CBHW080847020526
44107CB00080B/2661